The Human Repair Manual

by Dr. Mark Sexton N.D., PhD.

Models covered
All makes, models and years

Table of Contents

Exploded view

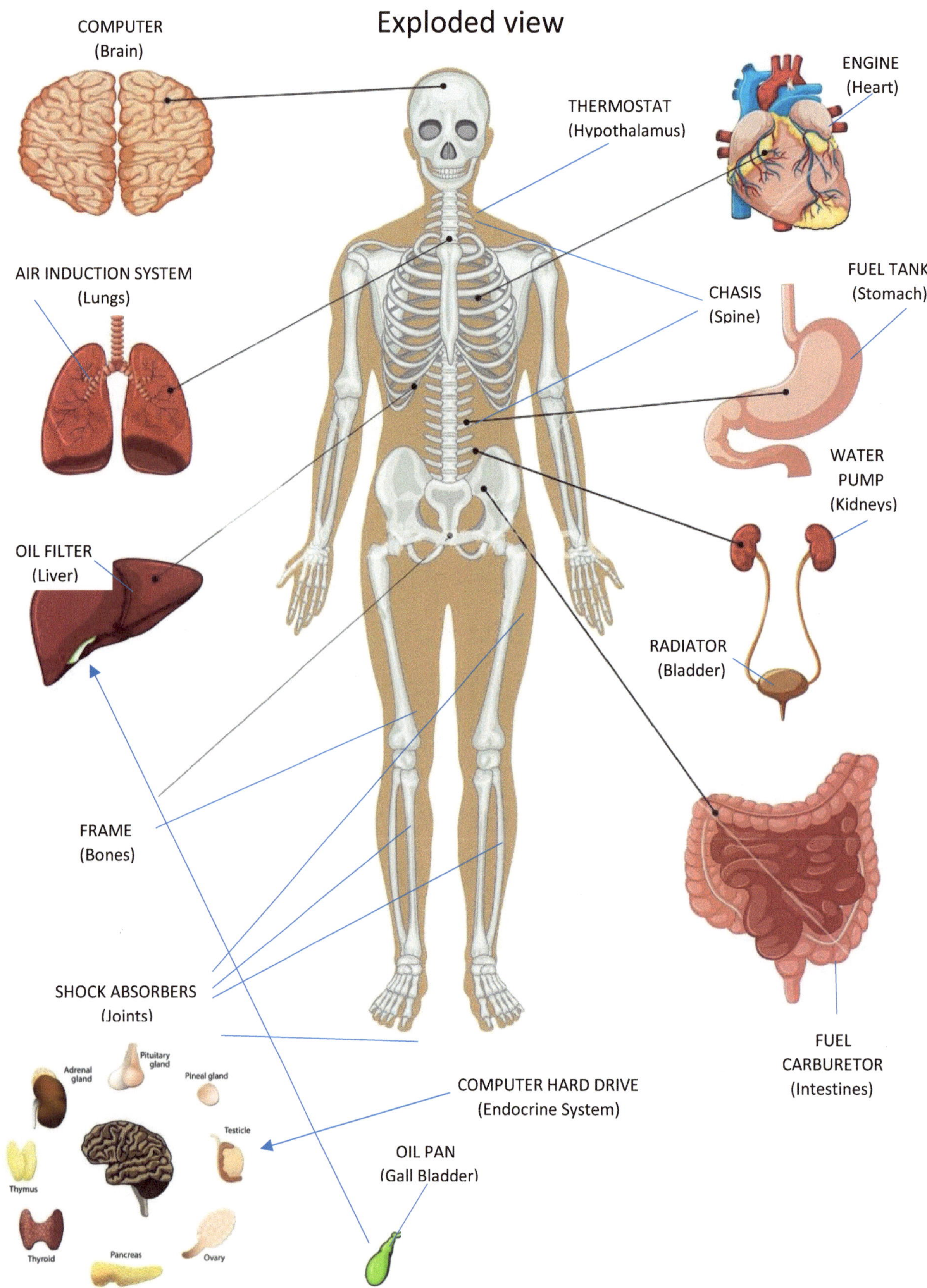

Chapter 1 GETTING STARTED

Contents

Purpose of this book
Tool Box
Systems Approach
Vehicle Overview
Broken Parts
Myths
Summary

Purpose

What is the purpose of this book? To provide a concise and simplified set of rules and guidelines to easily heal your body of most illnesses and maintain a healthy state of existence for the absolute optimal length of time possible. In simplified mechanic talk, "Make this sucker run like a bat outta hell 'til her wheels fall off!"

When you look under the hood of a car, you find many similarities with the human body.

You will discover a Battery,(the heart,) fuel filter (kidneys), computer (the brain) wires (the nervous system), fuel system, (digestive system) hoses, (the circulatory system), lymphatic system, immune system, (diagnostic sensing devices), frame work (bones), muscles (body design), paint (skin.)

TOOL BOX

Unlike for car maintenance, only a limited number of tools will be needed for maintaining the human machine.

THE BASICS

1. Alkaline water (Made with a machine or adding Baking Soda) for hydration and voltage.
2. 90 specific nutrients (Minerals, vitamins, amino acids and EFA's "essential-fatty-acids.") these are the crucial building blocks for the body to function, rebuild and repair.
3. Oxygen- crucial for cellular function and healing.
4. Exercise- to create voltage

All the tools will be discussed in greater detail as we go along with specialty tools being explained when needed for specific problems.

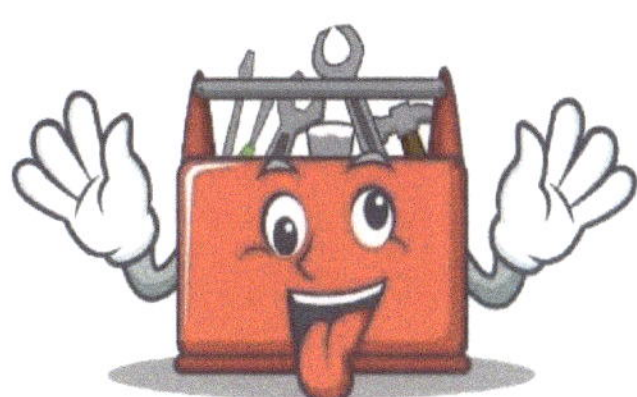

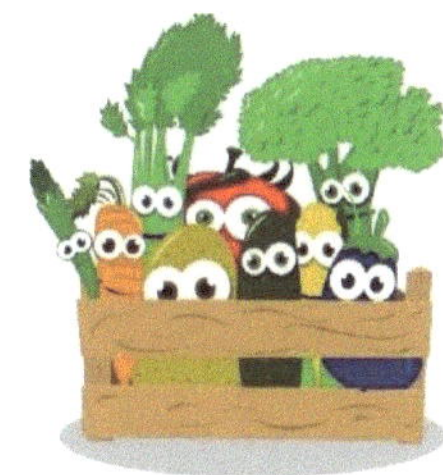

First, we're going to cover the basics of maintaining the human machine before we get into the diagnostics and actual repair work. We will finish off with a maintenance program that will give you the optimal mileage and performance you desire as when selecting a fine automobile. After all, you want this human vehicle to last a lifetime..

VEHICLE OVERVIEW

Let's start with an overview of the human body and a general and simplified explanation of how it works. To start with, we have, on the average, depending on size, 70 to 75 trillion cells that make up your body. And interestingly enough, and remember this, <u>it was started from one single cell</u>. This means your body knows how to heal itself. You don't need a master mechanic to keep it running. As you will see, healing the human body of most maladies including high blood pressure, asthma, diabetes and even some more serious, is quite simple and in many cases, fairly rapid.

Even incurables and so called "genetic" illness can be significantly improved upon if not totally eradicated by expanding our knowledge a little and following a few simple guidelines. The <u>Grand Illusion</u> that it takes lots of sophisticated and expensive equipment to heal the human body has been greatly exaggerated to sell more pharmaceutical drugs. Our illnesses are not caused by a deficiency in drugs. Now, this is not a manual for bashing the medical industry, as they do perform some amazing feats. So, this is all I am going to say on that subject. Except, I wish they would lighten up and open their minds to alternative treatments. This was the mainstream medicine that worked over 100 years ago and we are all STILL the same organic body that we were 100 years ago.

BROKEN PARTS   (How Disease Begins)

<u>THE NUMBER 1 MOST IMPORTANT RULE</u>:

"Disease begins ONLY when your body stops making healthy cells that work."

Every 6 months every cell in your body has been replaced. However, the key here is, the new cell can only be produced to the same health degree as the mother. So, we must repair, heal and strengthen the mother cells by cleaning out the toxins and provide the essential building blocks to repeatedly birth healthier cells through each new generation, until all cells reach ultimate potential. Now, we have restored our health and returned our body's condition to nearly assembly-line perfect, if not better.

Staying healthy means: removing accumulative toxins, keeping your pH's (voltages) in correct range, supplying water oxygen and the 90 nutrient building blocks needed. (More on pH's later on in the manual) We will go more into nutrition as we go on, as well.

<u>VERY IMPORTANT TO REMEMBER</u>:

Barring any structural defect you may have been born with, unless you actually get bit by some uninvited sucker carrying a germ such as malaria, typhoid or ingest salmonella from an unfit food source, "any illness you contraindicate during your whole visit on this planet will be caused by toxins." That's right. From poor dietary choices, environmental pollutants or lifestyle choices, toxins cause 90% of ALL illnesses. Now, I'm not saying your lifestyle choices are necessarily bad ones. I'm saying that the specific job or surroundings you work in may be subjecting you to toxin exposure.

MYTHS

Let's clear up a few myths that have been circulating since the beginning of the first genome study.

Did you know: it has been estimated that only 4% of ALL diseases blamed on genetics, are indeed genetic related? Now, mind you, there are such circumstances known as "inherent weaknesses" but this doesn't mean you are destined to suffer from a debilitating disease. We find our weaknesses to gain new strength.

Did you know: genes do not possess the ability to turn themselves "ON" or turn themselves "OFF"? They have to have an outside stimulant and that stimulant is usually, you guessed it…TOXINS! As long as you know the possibility of the weakness, you can strengthen that system or organ and prevent any occurrence that any family member down the bloodline may have experienced.

Most people do not inherit a weakness, <u>they inherit a diet</u>. You have heard someone say, "Everyone in my family inherited heart disease or diabetes or blah, blah, blah." No, what they inherited was a diet. A poor diet! This is very important to remember and to repeat to yourself. This is your mantra to recite whenever some unknowledgeable person starts trying to fill your ears with nonsense about aunt so and so or uncle Bob that had his leg amputated because of…? IT never had to be that way. Mantra: "I control my health and my destiny. <u>I</u> choose how healthy I want to be. No one else!"

Did you know: you can program your cells to heal your body? There is a Universal Law that says, *"Energy follows Intent."* This means, anything you want to happen in your life, you can make happen, simply by stating it to be and truly believing it WILL be. This includes healing. Now, I would not rely totally on this law while continuing to abuse your machine with garbage because, through the laws of "cause and effect," the fact you might not be not taking care of your human automobile, is much like your parents observing your responsibility, or lack of, with their car. If you don't show you are responsible and serious about your vehicle, you will not receive the performance and longevity desired. I will stop with that before I get too ethereal. You can buy one of my up and coming manuals on that subject. But remember, before any thought leaves your mind, good or bad, it travels down through and programs every one of your 70 trillion cells, good or bad. Then, they begin programming your environment as they exit your cells and begin to materialize. "Energy follows intent." Remember that.

OVERVIEW IN SUMMARY

You only need to follow a simple guideline and maintenance program to enjoy years of quality service. You will find, by following these simple rules, how easy it is to heal the human body from the simplest to the most chronic, incurable and genetic-referred illnesses, without having millions of dollars' worth of diagnostic equipment and a huge staff of college-trained personnel. Your body knows exactly what it needs and how to utilize those needs to repair anything wrong with it if given the chance and ingredients. Grant it, given the condition of the disease and the response time of the person, some conditions may take longer than others, but most symptoms and illnesses will be all but, if not totally eradicated, by the time a full body detox is performed, including high blood pressure and blood sugar levels. The FULL BODY DETOX (Tune-up) will be discussed in detail towards the end of the manual.

Chapter 2   SCHEMATICS and BLUPRINTS (DNA)

Contents

SCHEMATICS AND BLUEPRINTS   (DNA)

Now, when your body rolled off the assembly line, it was designed with a blueprint or DNA. This program stays with you throughout the entire length of stay. It is programmed for perfection. If for some reason, there are flaws, more likely than not, humans got in the way of nature. Nature, for the most part, DOES NOT make mistakes. If you trace the trail back far enough, you will find an intervention of human negligence, be it toxins from foods, drugs, pharmaceuticals, vaccines or environmental pollutants. Again, keep in mind, your body produced itself from one single cell. It knows, better than any mechanic, how to repair itself. Sometimes your computer becomes scrambled with toxins and their attached negative electrical frequencies, and needs wiped clean just like your computer hard drive.

FIXING BROKEN PARTS   (Herring's Law)

It's very important to know, "The body heals itself from the inside out and from top to bottom, in that order." This is known as "Herring's Law." This means the deepest inset illnesses will be dealt with first and the rest will follow in order of importance. The coolest thing is, unlike a car, you need only to have a select amount of tools and not have to bust your knuckles to keep it at optimal performance level.

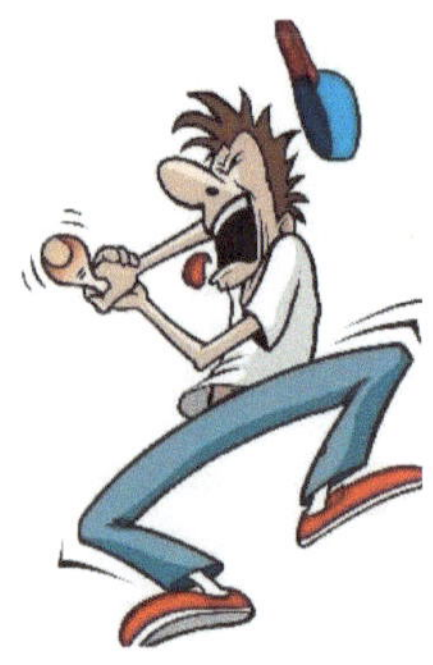

THE MECHANICS OF DNA

DNA is cool. It stands for "deoxyribose nucleic acid." It's a mouthful. Its such a complicated substance but in actuality, its ingredients are quite limited. It's made up of 4 amino acids: adenine, guanine, cytosine and thymine. Now, there are approximately 3 billion combinations that can be made with these 4 ingredients and they are called "bases." Strangely enough, 99% of all the bases found in humans are identical. That means even in the physical, we are nearly 'One in the Same." Someday, we'll get that! Now, if you add sugar "D-ribose sugar," (you can actually buy this stuff online and eat it) and phosphate to the "base," you have a DNA double stranded, twisting Helix worm that forms the physical bases of all life.

Another cool thing about DNA: when cells divide, they need an instructional building manual so, the DNA simple makes a copy of itself. Now, all that information is downloaded to the cell just like email.

RNA

There's another similar substance that works hand in hand with DNA that's called "RNA" or "Ribonucleic acid." It is basically a xerox copy of the original DNA blueprint, only in smaller sections. For instance, when the exterior "perceiver" antennas (or preceptor-sites)of a cell detect an intruder, such as a flu virus, they send a message to the receivers on the inside (or receptor-sites), that we need an antigen or antidote to kill the intruder. Here's the cool part. A protein key unlocks and opens the tool box of cellular DNA and an RNA remedy is created by copying the selected DNA base combinations. Virus gone! This type of action/reaction goes on in every cell of your body every moment and every day of your life and the life of the cell.

INTERESTING STORY: A DNA scientist performed a study by testing or analyzing the DNA of every living creature he could find to work with. He isolated the one strand of DNA that was common to ALL life forms in his researched. In other words, there is one DNA strand that every living creature he tested shares. Next, he analyzed and isolated DNA backwards down the line until he found the one and only species that was made up "solely" of this one DNA strand common to all species. It has NO other DNA strand in its makeup. This means, for the most part, ALL other species of life forms are related to this one species. Do you know what that one species happens to be.....? a SEA SPONGE. The sea sponge is comprised solely of the one DNA strand prevalent in all living things. Does this mean we are ALL related to Sponge Bob?

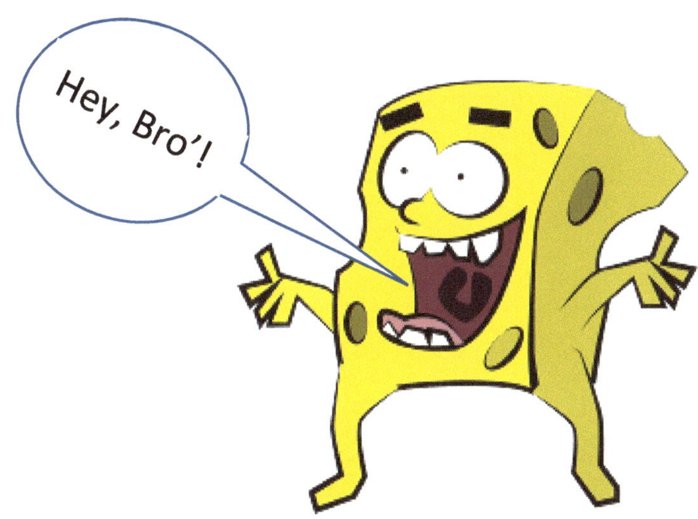

CHAPTER 3 ENGINE OVERVIEW

Contents

Engine Parts

 Just as the engine in your car is comprised of many parts and systems, your human engine is made up in much the same way. Both your car engine and your body burn fuel that results in the production of "kinetic energy" or (movement.) Both systems manufacture heat and residue in the process that must be released and removed by means of specifically designated systems and the two are very closely related as you will soon begin to discover.

Here is a breakdown and comparative similarities of our car vs human engine.

Valves and Pistons- Heart

This baby runs night and day, beating 115,000 times a day. That's about 60 rpm at idle speed and can rev out at 200 rpm 288,000 beats a day when the gas is applied to the floor. Of course, running full out for long periods is a way to blow your engine. Red line is about 260 rpm. Get ready to throw a rod or bust a valve at those rpm's.

Carburetor- The intestines.

This is where the fuel is injected, from the gas tank (stomach) mixed and distributed for usage throughout the vehicle.

Alternator- Cell Mitochondria

These are little powerhouse generators within each cell that turn nutrients into battery energy.

Voltage Regulator- Cells

Your cells are constantly adjusting and regulating your voltages or (pH's)

Water Pump- Kidneys

Water regulator and filtration system.

Thermostat- Hypothalamus

Constantly regulates engine running temperature.

Exhaust Manifold and Exhaust System- Kidneys, Lungs, Intestines, Skin, Intestines

This is the system responsible for removal of spent fuel bi-products or waste. Just like your car, the release of the fuel by-product exhaust prevents back pressure in the engine. If too much pressure is allowed to build up in the human vehicle, a turbo charger must be brought in to aid in relieving this backpressure. This would be called "A laxative." Epsom Salts can blow out an exhaust system like a cherry bomb in a school commode!

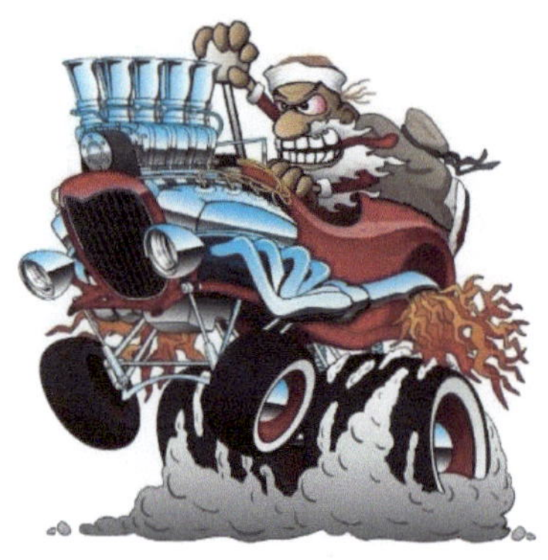

Chapter 4   FUEL SYSTEM (Digestive System)

Contents

FUEL GRADE

To start with, just like your automobile, for optimal mileage and overall performance, you want to ingest the highest-grade fuel you can obtain. This doesn't mean go to the grocery store and buy the most expensive items on the shelf. This means, look for the cleanest ingredients, devoid of chemicals like food colorings, preservatives and genetic modification (GMO) and try to buy organic. Well worth it.

COMBUSTION vs VOLTAGE

Just as your combustible engine in your car relies on controlled intermittent fuel explosions to create propulsion, your body too, relies on fuel explosions. There is only a slight difference in the two. The gasoline explosions creates combustive force and exhaust residue. Whereas, the explosion of your food fuel, creates electricity or voltage and the residue is referred to as ash. Very similar to the residue left by burning a piece of wood. The new important observation to start making, "is it "acid" or "alkaline" ash?

What creates this explosion? Your digestive enzymes colliding with the enzymes in the newly consumed food. Now, if your digestive enzymes are not optimal, you will not obtain the performance, power or mileage you are expecting. If they are, look out! You will generate electrical power to spare.

OVERHEATED FUEL

There is another element in this equation to be factored in: If the food is over-cooked (past 180 degrees) its enzymes are destroyed and there will be no explosion. You want electricity to be generated in every bite of food. Again, this is accomplished by the digestive enzymes of the food smacking into the digestive enzymes produced by your pancreas and liver. Now, if your liver enzymes are too weak, there will be no explosion. This is stated as "energy IN is greater than energy OUT. More on that subject when we get to the "oil filter" (liver) section.

Rule #1: "You DO NOT live on the food you eat. You live on the "energy" created by the digestion of the food you eat." You are electric.

FUEL DIAGNOSTICS   (Lymphatic and Immune System)

Did you know: that 75% of your immune system is located over your intestines and 60% of your lymphatic system is located there as well? These guys are constantly diagnosing and analyzing our fuel quality. This is the greatest clue that "what we eat determines the health of our bodies." Would you deliberately put gas in your car with dirt, debris and inferior ingredients, depriving you of the maximum performance out of your automobile? What would you do if you were told, this were the one and only automobile you will ever receive your whole life? Get the picture? Would you not take the greatest of care for this automobile, especially if your life depended on it?

When we subsidize or diet with sodas, chips, fried, refined foods and toxins, we are not only filling our human vehicle with sludge in our fuel, we are depriving it of the vital ingredients needed to perform, period; let alone performing at an optimal level. With poor being your choice of fuel, expect poor gas mileage and frequent breakdowns with a huge decrease in horsepower. Your body needs 90 high quality essential nutrients, water, oxygen and exercise for voltage to function properly and optimally. Better gas, better car, longer life expectancy. No reason for this sucker not to run way past its warranty.

EMISSION CONTROL (Allergies)

Every morsel of food going into the digestive system is inspected by the 75% of the immune system, as mentioned earlier, before being allowed to pass through or be rejected and sent back into the system. If a large quantity or as with many, most of the food particles coming in are rejected as unfit for use, the immune system goes into a state of "hyper-activity", rejecting everything it comes in contact with. In this situation a cat can walk across your yard. You never eat the cat, but now, you are allergic to cats. You merely looked at the cat, but your eyes are preceptor sites, also hooked to the immune system. It triggered an allergen alert.

This is how your body knows what digestive enzymes it needs to start preparing, even before the food enters your mouth. The eyeballs, the windows to the soul are also undercover spies for the immune system. They are telling on you.

Every cell in your body has hundreds of preceptor-sites or antennas, on the outside of the cell's membrane, constantly monitoring the environmental surroundings. When an intruder moseys along, the preceptors on the outside, send a message to receptors on the inside to make an antigen to destroy the intruder.

Now, if your body is full of sludge and the immune system is wading through muck, it will not be able to do its job adequately. The allergen may just be able to slip by unnoticed.

METHOD OF REPAIR:

" Full Body Detox", allowing the immune system to calm back down.

Remove all possible allergen-related foods, again, allowing for the immune system to balance.

Refrain from dairy and gluten, possibly forever. Try re-introducing these slowly, if you must.

TOOLS NEEDED:

B-Complex- 100 mg of each major B vitamin daily.

Acidophilus- Highest dosage you can find. Take once or twice daily.

Digestive enzymes- with each meal

Chapter 5 ELECTRICAL SYSTEM

Contents

COMPUTER   (Brain)

The brain is the main control center for the body. It computes, delegates, analyzes, regulates and oversees the entire operation of the human body. Some may wonder is it a muscle or an organ. It is sometimes referred to as the thinking muscle, but its actually and organ.

Weighing in at an average of 3 pounds. By weight its 50% cholesterol. It also contains 25% of the total cholesterol in your body as well as requiring 20% of the body's oxygen. Your brain retains 60% of the total amount of blood in your body at any given time. Your brain also has tiny hair-sized vessels supplying its blood. These vessels are so small, how small are they? They are so small; the blood corpuscles must enter in single file or they cannot pass through.

If your brain does not receive enough blood, oxygen or nutrients, it begins to shrink. Hence, you now have the beginning of Alzheimer's' Disease, which is shrinking of the brain. How so, you might ask? And I'm glad you did ask that question. Every blood corpuscle contains 4 oxygen molecules, as well as the vital nutrients needed specifically by the brain. Now, if your blood becomes thickened or sticky, the blood cannot pass through single file and begins clogging up these tiny vessels. Leave a tourniquet on a body part and see how long before it shrinks from lack of blood flow.

What causes thick blood? I'm glad you asked that question too.

1. If your body becomes too acidic, your blood becomes sticky.
2. If your blood sugar spikes or drops, your blood becomes thick.
3. If you have too much salt in your body, your blood becomes thick.
4. If you do not digest and assimilate animal protein well, your nitrates or ammonia levels rise, due to unprocessed protein and this can make your blood become thick very quickly. This can even cause hallucinations when allowed to climb too high and this can lead to immediate heart shut down.

Interesting fact about the brain: There have been people found to contain only a half dollar sized amount of gray matter in the front portion of the skull. The rest of the skull was hollow. These persons all showed signs of high intellectuality.

Interesting fact # 2: When up to 80% of a human brain has been removed, the person still retains full memory capacity, lending fact to the idea that the memory is stored in the cells that make up the body. Makes sense, as every cell in our body responds to thought and suggestions.

BATTERY   (HEART)

The heart has multi-representations in this manual from engine, to battery, to cooling system pump and oil pump. As you will see, it serves many functions.

The average weight of a human heart is 11 oz. Way less than a car battery. It beats approximately 115,000 times a day. It comes complete with a set of valves and pistons. It is made up of three main compartments and has attached to it over 6000 miles of vessels which we will refer to as hoses. It even comes with its own self-contained electrical system called the "cardiac conductor system." It's ALL about electricity.

Do you know what the one and only element of the human that determines if you are alive or dead? The one and only element that can make you alive again if you are dead? Electricity!

When you die, electricity is applied and if your battery (heart) is good enough to hold a charge, you're alive again. Think about that. Its ALL about electricity. Your car is probably on a 12 VOLT electrical system. If it is not of the correct voltage, say if your alternator is not charging well or your battery is weak, your car will lose some of its functions or may not work at all. This is not much different than our human machine. Only big difference is our bodies run on a 7.4 pH system or -22.5 mV. (millivolts)

Just as every other system in your body repairs itself during times of rest, your heart actually performs repairs in between beats, similar to your battery recharging during rest periods.

VOLTAGE REGULATOR   (CELLS) pH's and Voltage

The total voltage of the human body averages 3.5 trillion volts. With potential of up to 70 trillion volts generating capacity. Each cell membrane potential is .07 volts or 70 mV (hundredths of a volt)

Mind you, cells are not all activated simultaneously, but if they were all to turn on full blast at once, you would radiate like a search light.

The "Aura" is the accumulative sum of all the energy we produce. The more energy you are producing, the stronger your aura radiates. More on that in the chapter under Radio Frequency Adjustments.

Cells are designed to run between 7.35 pH which is (-20 mV) to 7.45pH which is (-25 mV)

Its ALL about *electricity*. This is what we are. We are electrical light beings navigating a physical, organic vessel. And the electrical frequencies must be correct for each area of the body, down to each individual cell.

Voltage: Understanding of

A BRIEF OVERVIEW OF pH's or Voltage

pH stands for "potential hydrogen." We are in essence measuring the amount of hydrogen atoms present or absent from the substance being measured.

The pH chart goes from 0 pH being the most acidic to 14 pH being the most alkaline. 7.0 pH being neutral. Neutral is the pH most drinking water is kept at.

Anything below 7 is acidic

Anything above 7 is alkaline.

pH is also a measurement of voltage. It is very important to know the references to pH and voltages are interchangeable. If the pH changes, the voltages change accordingly.

It is also important to understand; Alkaline pH is negative -mV whereas, Acid pH is positive +mV.

A pH chart is provided in the index at the back of this manual.

Now that we know a little about pH's let's see how they are applied and react in our human vehicle's machinery.

Making new cells requires -
1. 50 millivolts of energy (7.88 pH)
2. Amino Acids for the insides of the cells
3. Fats to make the outside of the cells (remember this, the outside membrane of the cell is fats)
4. Vitamins and Minerals to make the metabolic process work (90 specific ones)
5. Oxygen
6. Fats and Glucose for fuel

When we lose electrons, we lose voltage. Another way put: when a cell becomes acidic, it has lost electrons. pH down, voltage down. This causes disease.

When your voltage is low, your organs simply don't have the horsepower to do their job.

Voltage Loss

Electron stealers-
Anything below 7.0 pH
Acid water- 0 -6.9pH
Free Radicals- are molecules missing electrons (these are positive poles)
Pharmaceutical medicines- acidic
Moving wind- This is why riding in a convertible wears you out. Sleeping under a fan makes you tired. Air conditioning, hair dryers all make you tired.
Still water- taking a bath makes you tired compared to a running shower that stimulates.
Fluoride- water , toothpaste, medicines, etc.
Processed sugars-acidic
Alcohol and tobacco products-acid
Carbonated Beverages-acid
Processed foods
Caffeinated beverages-pop, coffee, tea, etc.-all acid

"Kirchoff's Law of Voltage" put simply, states, *"An area of high voltage causes electrons to flow to an area of low voltage."*

Voltage Gain

Electron Donors
Anything above 7.0 pH.
Alkaline water
Alkaline fruits and vegetables
Hugs- transfer electrons from one individual to another. (High voltage to low voltage electron transfer "Kirchhoff's Law of Voltage")

<u>Animal petting</u>- they are very high voltage beings. By touching or holding them, their high voltage replenishes our low voltage with electrons.

<u>Walking on the Earth barefoot</u>- We all know walking barefoot in the grass makes up feel less stressed, more peaceful and grounded. No human being on the planet can match the voltage of the Earth. You will definitely reap the benefits of the electron transferring effect.

<u>Hugging a tree</u>- Again, their voltage is always higher than a human's, as they are rooted to the earth. The electrons are transferred to us from the Earth via the tree.

<u>Moving Water</u>- This is why swimming in the ocean makes you invigorated, as does taking a shower. Baths make you tired (still water)

<u>Exercise</u>- Moving muscles create electrons. This is a major way the body acquires electrons. Exercise invigorates.

<u>Craniosacral pump</u>- when activated, sends a surge of electrons through our body.

<u>Anti-Oxidants</u>- These are anything that donates free electrons, i.e., blueberries, Goji berries, vitamin C, Vitamin E, hugs, trees, etc.

Note: The higher the voltage of water, the more oxygen that will be dissolved making a higher oxygenated water. Voltage drop causes oxygen to come out of solution.

Note: When oxygen is available, for every unit of fatty acids, we create 38 molecules of ATP (cell energy). However, if oxygen is unavailable, only 2 units
of ATP (cell energy) are created. We went from 38 miles to the gallon to 2 miles per gallon.

Note: When injured, the injured area's voltage immediately goes to -50 mV to begin healing and generating new cells. At -50 mV, there is pulsing pain due to high voltage.

Fact: When you hurt ALL the time, you have LOW voltage.

Note: When voltage drops to +30 mV or 6.48 pH cancer can develop.
The human body has thousands of live fungus, viruses and bacteria lying dormant waiting for the opportunity to wake up. Acid does just that.
It fertilizes these pathogens like Miracle Grow on plants. They want food. What food do they want? Your cells. Your electrons. If you are acidic, you're lunch.

Note: Emotions can affect our pH levels. When we get angry, sad or upset, our pH can drop 2-5 points in a matter of seconds.

Producing Voltage

HOW DO CELLS GET VOLTAGE?
1. Live organic foods- they still have life and contain minerals that create voltage.
2. Minerals- The higher voltage, alkalizing minerals are Potassium, Magnesium, Calcium and sodium. Potassium and Calcium are used to make alkaline water.
3. Alkaline water-contains alkalizing minerals (Potassium and calcium + others)
4. Exercise- your muscles are electron pumps. Each time you move, you are creating voltage.
SO MOVE!

CELLS NEED THESE TO BE HEALTHY

Cell membranes are made of fat. (GOOD FAT)
1. Water with voltage (Alkaline water)
2. Fats to make cell membranes
3. Amino acids to make the "cytoplasm" (the machinery) inside the cell.
4. Vitamins to allow the body to make fats and proteins work.
5. Minerals to make the fats and proteins work and to keep your pH's in the operating range.
6. Oxygen
7. Sunshine
8. The body must have voltage (alkaline pH) to function. 7.35 to 7.45 pH which means the same as -20 mV to -25 mV

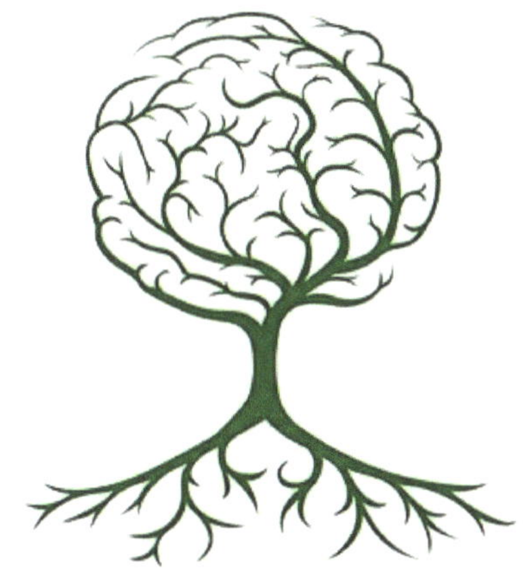

Hug the Earth
get a brain electron
transfer

Chapter 6 RADIO FREQUENCY ADJUSTMENT (Electrical Frequency Tuning)

Contents

Hertz

Hertz

Look at your body as a radio and each individual organ and system therein, a radio station. When you begin treating and repairing the human vehicle, you are merely adjusting and tweaking electrical frequencies or tuning in the various radio stations into their proper frequency range. For instance, your pancreas should be operating on a frequency of 4.9 Hertz or "cycles per second." When the pancreas becomes overworked, it begins to fade out of its ideal frequency range. When its slips down to 3.0 Hertz or 2.5 Hertz, the pancreas is now at an inability to function and so the beginning of diabetes. With continued abuse, you move into the full-blown diabetes syndrome.

For those of you who might not know what a "Hertz" is, or an electrical "frequency", I will explain. The two terminologies are inner changeable. Another way to phrase it is "cycles per second." The term "hertz" refers to a sine wave's pattern, during a 1 second interval, traveling from neutral to positive, then to negative and back to the neutral beginning point. In other words a hertz or frequency is the number of times a sine wave performs this pattern in one second. Hence, 10 hertz would be the sine wave repeating this pattern 10 times in one second. (Below, see the two up/down humps? 2 Hertz, 1 second.)   The sine wave has made two complete cycles. 2 Hertz or 2 cycles per second.

Sine wave (2 Hertz/cycles, in 1 second interval)

Radio Adjusting Insight

Now, that we have a basic understanding of a Hertz, we will dive into tweaking the radios of our vehicle. You will see, this is truly what we are always doing when healing or repairing the body.

Referring, once again, to the "Aura" mentioned in the last chapter; The aura is simply the sum of ALL the electricity being generated within the human body and just like a light bulb, we generate more than can be contained, so it radiates outward.

If you were to sense a darker spot in an area of the aura, you could trace that spot down the coinciding meridians to the organs or system/s lying along that meridian line, boost the correct frequency using electricity, color or sound and the dark spot will disappear, as the frequencies are restored and the aura once again in balance or harmony..

When we take a supplement, let's say vitamin C for instance, we are not taking the vitamin C to obtain the compounds in the vitamin C. We are taking the vitamin C to receive the electrical frequencies attached to each molecule that makes up the compound of vitamin C.

We get vitamin D through the sunlight. Do you see vitamin capsules floating through the air? Of course not. It's ALL electrical frequencies. The "Zen" of the human body, its very nucleus, is electricity in many specific frequency ranges. This is why it is important to understand this information. When we realize this, we understand the simplicity of healing this incredibly intricate vehicle we call "human beings." It sounds so simple to be true, but it is! It is both simple and true.

Correcting Frequency Interference

So, remembering each cell, each organ, each system in the human body has specific frequency ranges for optimal health, and toxins have now been introduced into the system. These toxins have electrical frequencies attached to them as well. The problem here being, they (toxins) are of the wrong frequencies and begin to interfere with the correct healthy frequencies of your radio system.

Imagine trying to tune in your favorite radio station, but your tuner is not quite up to par and there are other radio stations so close in proximity, that you cannot tune your targeted station in because of the static from the other stations. Well, let's call those interfering stations, toxins. Toxins in the system, conflict and steal frequencies and power from your targeted radio station. Before long, there are so many toxic frequencies that without their physical removal and the repairing of your tuner, the reception just continues to worsen until you reach a point of total disgust and frustration. This is why it is necessary to periodically clean out the system of these toxic frequencies and debris so we may go on enjoying our vehicle and its perfectly tuned radio system.

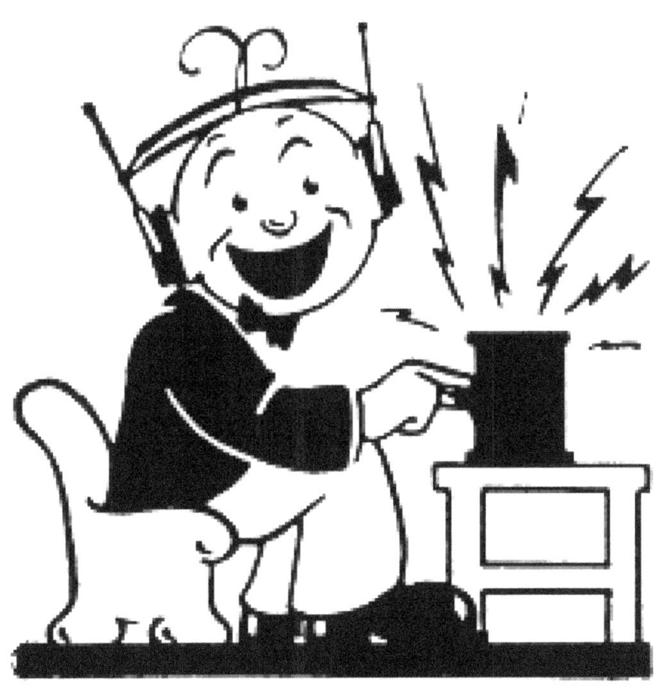

Chapter 7   OIL FILTER (Liver) OIL PAN (Gallbladder)

Contents

Oil Filter Overview

   Your liver has over 1000 specific functions and responsibilities to perform. Unlike your car oil filter, Your liver can't be replaced and must be flushed out periodically (approximately once a year unless you have been on medication or have eaten poorly for an extended period.) Then, by all means, flush it out.

   Your liver Is your blood filter as well as toxin remover, nutritional distribution center, immune system controller, food processor, enzyme producer and the liver contains over 35,000 square meters of membrane surface used to accomplish these feats. This membrane is made predominantly of fats.

   When you don't eat enough fat or eat fat that has been heated and processed into a plastic-like substance, the membranes don't work correctly. When the liver gets clogged with debris because the membranes are made of plastic, it tries to wash itself out with cholesterol.

   A "high cholesterol" level indicates the liver is trying to cleans itself or that it is trying to provide you with the raw materials of cholesterol-based hormones you are deficient in.

   If you interfere with the liver's natural process with drugs (Statin in particular) and continue to feed your body plastic cheeses and oils, you are doomed for a life of chronic illnesses of all types.

   Our liver synthesizes 1,500 – 2000 mg of cholesterol daily.

Note: If eating fats makes you nauseated, your liver isn't making enough bile to properly absorb them.

OIL FILTER FLUSH   *"Formula LF-1"*

LIVER FLUSH: The simplest way is placing ½ cup extra virgin olive oil + ½ cup fresh squeezed lemon juice in a mason jar. Shake and drink right before bed. Your liver will think its having a gallbladder attack and will produce 5 times more bile than normal. This will flush toxins, residue of medications and most other debris from the liver. This will occur about 3 A.M. in the morning and you will be totally unaware of the whole phenomenon.
   You can take it to more extremes and add coffee enemas to the maintenance regimen. This is done by brewing ¼ cup coffee and adding to 1quart distilled water. LET COOL! (This is a most important step to remember.) Next, place coffee mixture in a Fleets enema bottle and squirt up the rectum. Lie on your back for 15 minutes, left side 15 minutes, right side fifteen

minutes, then go to the toilet and expel. This may be done several times a week.

Interesting note: Each time you ingest extra virgin olive oil, you clean and detox the liver.

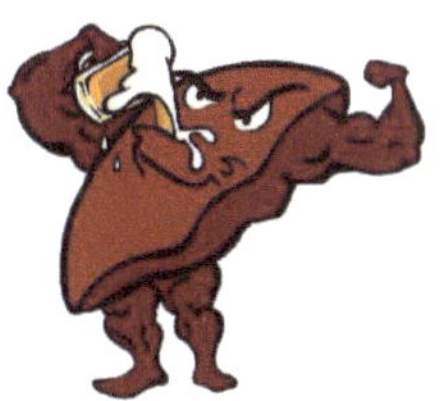

GALL BLADDER (Oil pan)

Your gallbladder is the storage facility for the liver produced bile.
Your liver makes approximately 3 cups of bile daily. Bile is used to extract the amino acids from the proteins in the stomach. It also dumps bile into the intestines every 3 1/2 hours.
The problem with gallbladder removal, your liver can't make bile fast enough for you to absorb the fat you need to keep healthy.

   What are gallstones? Another good question. Gallstones are made up of cholesterol. In the center of this cholesterol is the culprit. Unprocessed animal protein, which appears as sharp chards of glass that would slit your guts open if passed through your biliary tube and are coated with cholesterol by your liver, to prevent the gut slitting event from occurring.

Note: If you have had your gallbladder removed, you will have to take bile supplements the rest of your life. Or you will suffer greatly when eating fats.

Oil Pan Cleanout   *"Formula GBF-1"*

GALL BLADDER FLUSH: This is done to prevent or in many cases, eliminate gallbladder removal surgery. (Its well worth the try. This is generally done in conjunction with the Liver Flush, as they work synergistically.

Tools needed:
   Distilled water
   Unfiltered Apple juice
   Epsom Salts
   Lemons
   Extra virgin olive oil

PROCEDURE:
   1.Upon rising: Drink 1-quart distilled water.
   2.Next: Before noon, drink 1-quart unfiltered apple juice.
   3.For the remainder of the day until 5:00 p.m., drink nothing but distilled water.
   4.At 5:00 p.m.: mix 2 TBS Epsom Salt in 4 oz. distilled water w/the juice of ½ lemon.
     drink and chase with another quart of distilled water. (You should not leave your house

for the next few hours. This will expel all your new food. Very effectively.

5. Just before bed: Drink the above oil/lemon liver concoction.

6. Upon rising, drink 1 more TBS Epsom salt with same amount of water as before.
   You WILL expel gallstones in the next few hours. They will look like small meteorites
   and will be greenish or brownish in color. They will float, as they are made of.
   cholesterol which is very buoyant. They come out the south end, in case you were
   wondering and <u>pain-free</u> also, in case. Very similar to removing sludge from your gas.
   tank.

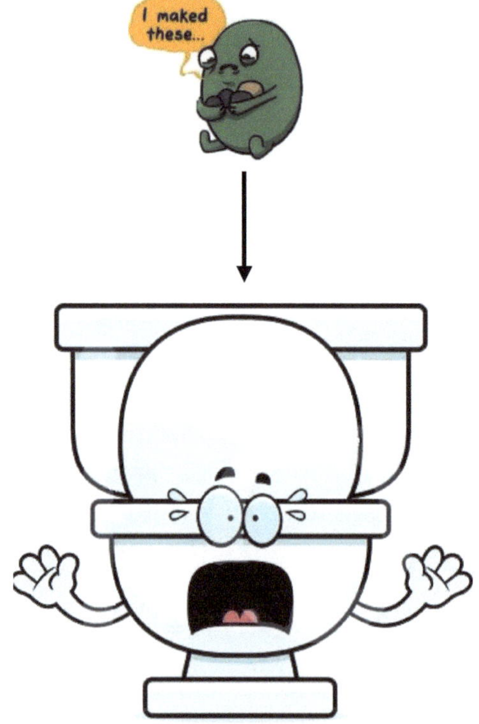

Later, Dude!

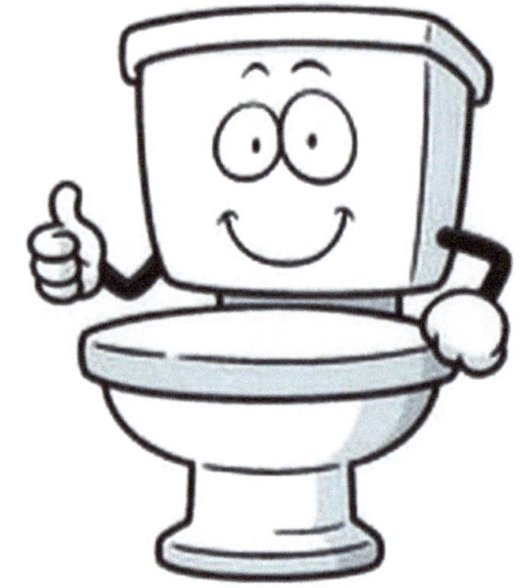

CHAPTER 8 TWEAKING FOR OPTIMAL ENGINE PERFORMANCE

Contents

Now, let's look over the different grades of fuels and the many additives we have to choose from to pour into our engines, and there are quite a few, some good and some not so good to down right "the worst crap you could put into your machinery."

VERY POOR-QUALITY FUEL ADDITIVES

These will definitely cause breakdowns in your vehicle.

Aspartame-

FACTS:

1. When heated past 92 degrees, it turns into formaldehyde. Our body temperature is 98.6 degrees. Formaldehyde is embalming fluid. It's for dead people, not living ones.

2. Some of its side effects are: cancer, seizures, symptoms mimicking MS, headaches, depression, ADHD, birth defects, Epilepsy, Lymphoma, Alzheimer's, Parkinson's, brain tumors and many more.

3. There is a 1500-page report of the bad side effects found associated with Aspartame, **ALL BAD**. Yet, Monsanto pushed its way thru anyway.

4. Aspartame is made from three ingredients: Aspartic Acid 40%, Phenylalanine 50%, Methanol 10%, (turns into formaldehyde, a neurotoxin that causes nerve and brain damage. The first two are both amino acids and very dangerous when not suspended in a protein, as is the case with Aspartame.

5. It turns to Formic Acid in a diabetic and begins eating the brain.

6. The World Health Organization put out a bulletin that 80% of ALL the case symptoms of MS would disappear in 2 weeks by stopping its usage.

7. Stay away from ALL artificial sweeteners. They are ALL Aspartame derivatives.

Food Colors- Unless labeled from natural sources, such as fruit or paprika, they are petroleum based and highly carcinogenic. If you see FD&C on the label, it means the FDA certifies it as a known carcinogen and you ingest it at your own risk. Good, healthy food in its natural state, needs no added food coloring. If it does, it's not natural. So don't eat it! **Anyway, this stuff will ruin your interior as well as stain your exterior.**

Preservatives- cause cancer and contribute to a large number of illness in this country. Most countries ban them from food usage.

HIGH QUALITY, HIGH PERFORMANCE ADDITIVES
(For specific and specialized needs.)

Liquid Vitamin/Mineral- supplement containing at least 90 nutrients. Intra-Max is a top recommendation. Contains 415 organic nutrients. Tastes good too.

Lysine- Great immune system booster.(1200 to 2500 mg daily)

Vitamin C- in Liposomal form- works perfect with Lysine. (up to 10,000 mg daily)

Omni-Immune- incredible immune booster. Will kill all mold, yeast, fungus, virus and bacteria present in your body.

Iodine- Anti-microbial and bactericide. Needed for thyroid hormones and brain development.
12.5 mg daily. If thyroid is hyper or hypo, you need 3x's this amount for 1-2 months.
Without proper iodine reserve, all the thyroid medication in the world will have little to no effect.

Phosphatidylserine- This is a supercharger for the brain. It will add clarity and much improvement in its performance. It may take 30-60 days before you notice anything, but when it kicks in…quarter mile in record time!

Astaxanthin- Strong heart, brain enhancer, used for Alzheimer's and Parkinson's diseases.

Liposomal Glutathione- If you have tremors or shaking in your suspension, this stuff works miracles. (Parkinson's and Alzheimer's.) Greatly improves mind function and restores clarity. 1-3 tsp daily. Redi-sorb.com or Livon Labs.com   I call these the "magic beans."

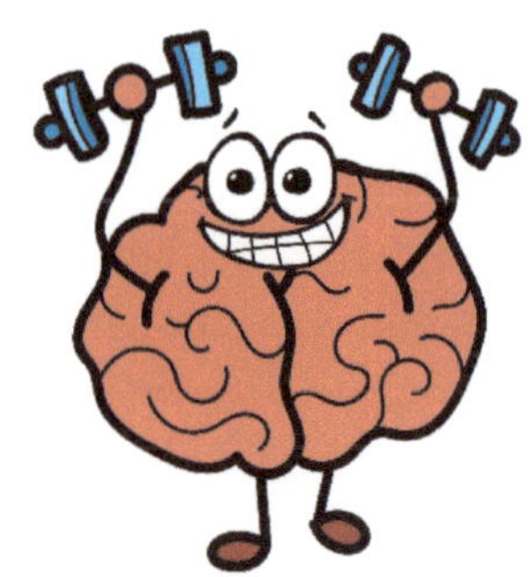

BRAIN STRONG!

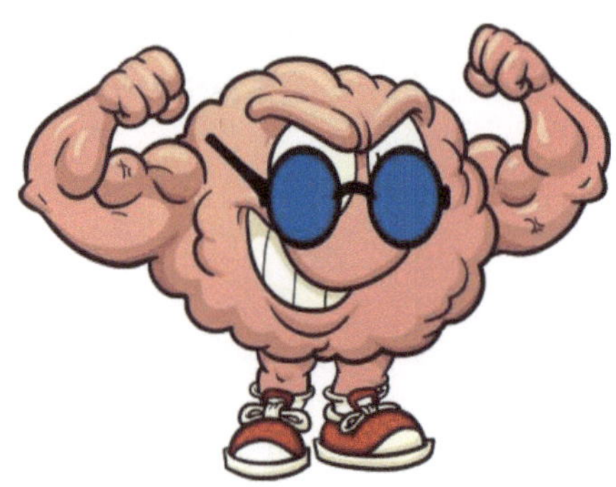

CHAPTER 9   OIL TECH 101

Contents

Like your car, periodically our bodies need a complete oil change. And like automobile oils, they come in a variety of weights and quality.

POOR QUALITY OILS AND THEIR SIDE EFFECTS

Hydrogenated or partially hydrogenated oils- Canola, corn oil, soy bean oil, coconut oil, whale oil.

1. These oils are heated to 350 degrees for 5 hours turning them into something similar to plastic.

2. When you eat these plastics, your cell membranes become plastic. When this happens, nothing can go in and nothing can come out. The cell sends out signals its hungry. In response, the body sends glucose and insulin to the cell. But it can't get through the plastic. Food is continuing to arrive on the scene without being eaten. The cell becomes surrounded in glucose and insulin but remains hungry. This is known as "insulin resistance" and type II diabetes. It eventually does the same exact thing to the brain made of plastic.

Canola Oil- (rapeseed) An industrial lubricant, 100% genetically engineered, considered a toxic and poisonous weed, causes lung cancer, insects won't even eat it.

Side effects include: loss of vision, disruption of nervous system, respiratory illness, anemia, increased heart disease, cancer, constipation, irritability and low birth weights in infants when the mother has ingested this toxic oil.

Studies have shown: Growth retardation, damage to heart muscles, lowered lung capacity and intolerance to colder temperatures.

In Europe, rapeseed was fed to cows, pigs and sheep and later went blind and started attacking people. No further attacks after rapeseed was eliminated.

Fried foods- These are ALL prepared in "trans-saturated fats" plastic membrane builders. Eat them for guaranteed degenerative diseases.

Restaurant cheeses- Same trans-fat oils that make up plastic membranes.

Margarine- Start with cheap oil, add Nickel Oxide (very toxic), add hydrogen gas in a very temperature oven, add emulsifiers to give it consistency. Next, it must be steamed cleaned at yet more high temps. As it is an unappetizing nasty gray color, it is then bleached and coal tar dyes and strong flavorings, added to make it resemble butter. Finally it is compressed and packaged, ready to eat and make all the plastic cell membranes you could ever desire. Your digestive system doesn't recognize trans-fats and incorporates them into cells.

Note: "Omega" is a heat tolerance factor. The higher the "Omega" the more heat the oil can take before breaking down. Very similar to the numbers on motor oils. 10-50 can take more heat before breaking down than 10-40 or 5-30.

Complete Oli Change Procedure

HOW TO CHANGE YOUR OIL

Discard any types of oils mentioned above.
Replace with Grade A organic Omega 9's for cooking.
Add Omega 3's (fish oils) and Omega 6's (flax oils) to your diet.
EFA's (essential fatty acids) 1200 to 2400 mg daily. Helps brain functions.

Note: EFA's increase absorption of vitamins and minerals, nourish hair, skin and nails, help produce hormones, ensure normal growth and development, aids in preventing and treating disease. Great for your brain.
Note: In changing your oil, you will replace the damaged plastic membranes of the cells with healthy, pliable, usable membranes. Healing is really that simple.

Engine Pollutants

WHAT ARE THESE CHEMICALS DOING TO ME?

Fluoride- is a waste by-product run-off from aluminum manufacturing plants. "Fluorine" is the mineral substance we have in our bodies, NOT fluoride. Fluoride is rated as a "neuro-toxin. It was never intended to be consumed by the human organism. The EPA has such an expensive method for disposal of fluoride, the lobbyists convinced the government it is a health additive to make your teeth and bones strong. So, they put it in our water supplies. They now make money disposing of it instead of the other way around.

Keep this in mind: <u>Iodine is the first element in the DNA sequence for human brain development.</u> Fluoride displaces iodine, leading to brain and neurological damage, damages collagen, allowing arteries to overstretch and rupture. This is a sure setup for heart disease. Tooth and bone deterioration are caused from consuming fluoride. It is poison to the human.

There are medications made from fluoride. Levaquin, Cipro , Celebrex, Flonase, Lipitor, Paxil, Prozac and many more. Several more Statin dugs contain fluoride.

When America came to the rescue to help the children of Africa, they began dropping like flies. After further investigation, it was discovered the kids were eating the toothpaste which contained enough fluoride (in one tube of toothpaste) to kill the children. If you notice on children's toothpaste it will usually say, "Do not allow to swallow."

The residue from fluoride, though filtered via the kidney's is still at half strength up to ten hours later. Fluoride accumulates in the body and is considered more toxic than lead but less than arsenic. Fluoride binds with magnesium creating an insoluble residue that deposits in the bones creating an extremely brittle bone condition easily fracture able. **"This crap will clog your pipes, brittle your suspension, short out your wiring and scramble your computer!"**

Note: Adolf Hitler ordered his scientists to find a substance to place in the drinking water that would suppress the rebellious nature in the human brain. They came up with Fluoride. They also found when too much was added to the water, people died. Stay away from the stuff!

Chlorine- A VERY TOXIC poison. It is used in bleach. Its used for killing living stuff. YOU are living stuff! Would you put acid down your gas tank? **It's a "Hole Burner." NO!**

Caffeine- Drives the adrenals into adrenal failure. Constricts blood vessels. One major causation of Erectile Disfunction. Bad on your shifter.

Processed sugars- Will lead to diabetes, weight gain, tooth decay, poor brain function.

Processed foods- Devoid of most original nutrients. Causation of many degenerative diseases.

Heavy Weight Oils

FATS AND CHOLESTEROL MYTH

About 20% of your body weight should be comprised of healthy fats since:

CHOLESTEROL

1. Your brain contains 25% of the total cholesterol in your body which averages out to about 2% of your total body weight, all being LDL. (The so called, "bad cholesterol.")
2. Your brain , by dry weight, is 50% cholesterol. (LDL)
3. Cholesterol is used to make ALL the hormones produced in the Adrenal Cortex. (LDL)
4. Sexual hormones, including testosterone, estrogen and progesterone are made from cholesterol. (LDL)

    Without it, sexual dysfunction occurs.

    Without it, brain and nerve disfunction occurs.

    Without it, liver backup occurs.

FATS

1. All of your cell membranes and most your nervous system is fat.
2. Saturated fats have gotten a bad rap because "plastic" fats are saturated.
3. Saturated fats are strong and unsaturated fats are porous.
4. Saturated fats make strong cells
5. Unsaturated fats make up the entrance and exits to the cells.
6. Animal fats are considered saturated, while fish, flax and olive oils are unsaturated.
7. The ratio between the two should be 4:1-Saturated to unsaturated. You should eat 4x's more saturated than un-saturated.
8. Mother's milk is extremely high in cholesterol, as it is essential for growth and development, fighting cancer, heart disease and mental illness.
9. Cholesterol keeps your arteries pliable. It actually saves you from heart attacks, not the other way around. Its what keeps your valves opening and closing.

STATIN DRUGS
The taking of cholesterol lowering drugs will prevent 1 death in 2000 person with cholesterol over 200 compared to no deaths in norm cholesterol.
This means there will be 1 additional death from higher cholesterol with drugs than persons with lower levels, per 2000 people and no drugs.
   You must have HDL as well as LDL ("bad cholesterol") cholesterol. Without LDL (bad cholesterol) your brain wouldn't function.
Cholesterol keeps you well and is produced by the liver. So what better way to keep people sick than to suppress the function of the liver?

   Its all an ongoing lie which started, non-intentionally, in the 1950's by a Dr. Keys, believing cholesterol causes strokes and heart disease. Upon retiring in 1997, Dr. Keys admitted **"There's no connection whatsoever between the cholesterol in food and blood cholesterol. None. And we have known this all along."**

Statin drug sales range around the tune of $1200.00 a year per person. Add to that the medications prescribed and sold for the side effects caused by the Statin drugs themselves.
It has been admitted: Statin drugs will cause a large percentage of Alzheimer's Disease. Why? Because we are using a synthetic chemical to stop the liver from doing its natural job.

Note: Your liver does not make cholesterol, but rather synthesizes it. Since cholesterol isn't water soluble, it cannot be suspended in the blood but must be carried by a protein called "lipo-proteins." Along with cholesterol, these proteins carry other fat molecules grouped in units of 3's.which are attached to "glycerol. Hence the name "triglycerides." The fats are carried and deposited in the liver. There, they are synthesized into **VLDL,** "very low density lipo-protein." The liver synthesizes between 1,500 and 2000 mg of **VLDL** daily. LDL is NOT "bad cholesterol." It is crucial to your health!

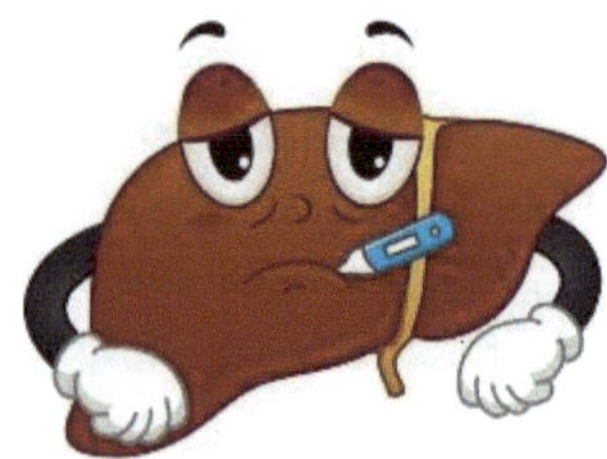

CHAPTER 10 - FUEL AND FUEL MIXTURES

Contents

Fuel Formula 6-2-1-1

Eat organic when possible.
The following mixture is based on your daily food intake. It is designed as an 80% alkaline diet. This will generate maximum voltage for your machine. Consider vegetables and fruits to be alkaline and proteins and starches, acidic. That said, here is the finest formula you can obtain for maximum performance, as well as excessive and sustainable energy.

"FORMULA 6-2-1-1"
(6 vegetables, 2 fruits, 1 protein, 1 starch)
Vegetables should be the bulk of your diet. About 60%
Fruits- should make up about 20%
Proteins (from animals)- should make up 10%
Starches- should be 10%
Meats- should be clean, antibiotic, growth hormone and steroid-free.
This designer formulation will keep your voltage right around -20mV or 7.4 pH.
(Perfect for cell function.)

Milk- In its RAW form has many health benefits and essential nutrients, though it still causes mucus formation and can attribute to allergies, asthma and sinus problems. When pasteurized and homogenized, it is no longer milk and anything but healthy and should be avoided at ALL costs.

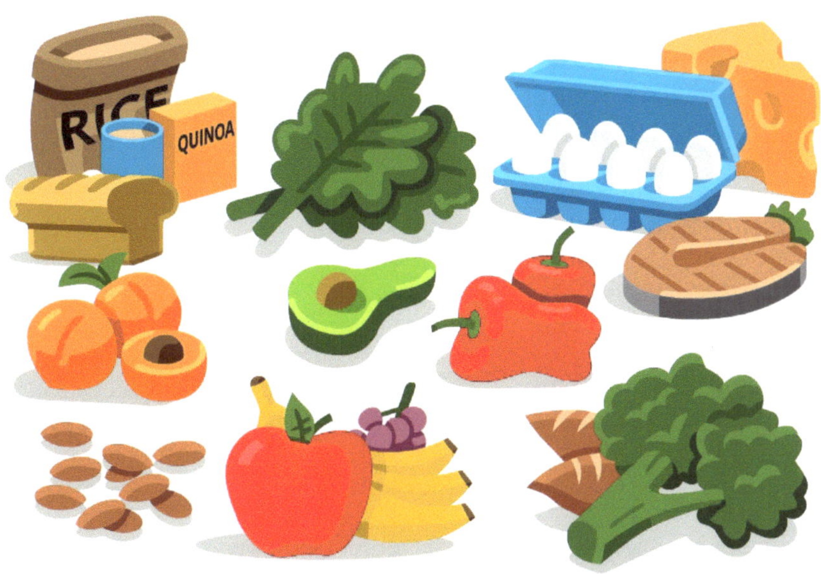

CHAPTER 11 SUSPENSION

Contents

Chassis Overview
Frame
Shock Absorbers
Potholes

Chassis Overview (spine)

The chassis is made up of 24 segments or hinges (vertebrae). Unlike the rigid car chassis, the human chassis is flexible, allowing movement while still lending support to the frame. There are disc-like pads between the hinges to cushion them from shock and protect them from friction wear. These are the "ball-joints" of the chassis.

As with the automobile, there is a chassis electrical system. There is a one main power cord going through the chassis as well as 31 pair of wires attached to the chassis that connect with the vast array of wires traveling to various parts and systems. So, besides providing structural support, the chassis acts as the "central bus-bar" as well. (Wire connection terminal)

The chassis can slip out of alignment, where upon we go see a chassis mechanic, or chiropractor. It is quite crucial to adjust the alignment as quickly as possible. The wires protruding from the chassis are nerves and each one is connected to a different area of the vehicle, similar to your cars fuse panel. The pain acts as your warning light that a fuse has blown.

When a fuse does get blown in the fuse panel, complications can arise, some quite serious Besides the obvious presence of pain, there can be many side effects from digestive problems to heart and lung complications.

When a section of the chassis slips out of alignment, wires may become pinched. As a result, there is a break in the electrical circuitry and that section will lose its connection to the central dispatcher.

Another complication with an out of alignment chassis is restriction of oil (blood) flow. Unobstructed oil flow is crucial for top performance.

Frame (skeleton)

There are 270 bones in your skeletal system at birth and decreasing to 206 by adulthood. Technically, there are also 6 additional **bones**, 3 in each ear, known as the ossicles. The frame or skeleton does more than just support our structure.
1 Offers an anchor for tendons and ligaments to aid in body movement.
2 Serves as an out protective shell for our inner organs
3 Bone marrow housing, the main source of blood formation or coolant for the human body.
4 It serves for a source of calcium for the entire body. This calcium helps alkalize the body from calcium out-of-balance diseases such as osteoporosis. Hence the hollowness in the bones, from extraction of calcium to alkalize the blood.

The composition of bone is 65% Hydroxyapatite, which is an insoluble salt of calcium and phosphorus, as well as small amounts of magnesium, sodium and bicarbonate. Water makes up about 25%
.
Strengthening the frame
While exercise will stimulate strength in the bones, there are a few additives that can be applied for extra strengthening:

Calcium, known as "The Knitter" is the main repair substance when we break a bone.(a Builder)
Both "**Strontium**" and "**Boron**" are amazing bone strengtheners.

Shock Absorbers (joints)

---

1   A joint is where two bones come together.
2   Your joints serve as shock absorbers.
3   ligaments serve as the connecting rods to hold the bones together.
4   Tendons connect muscle to bone.
5   Cartilage serves as the shock cushions at the end of the bones.

Joint Maintenance

EFA's (Essential Fatty Acids) act as lubricants for the joints

When the joints become creaky add some vitamin D3 and Calcium into the fluid.

Dehydration is another causation of creaky, cracking joints.

Pain in a joint may be deposited crystalized acids that need flushed with a Master Cleanse. (Found Under the tune-up section, Chapter 12.)

Suspension Maintenance and Precautions

Excessive Load Limits

Excessive weight will ruin your suspension (spine and bones) and shock absorbers. (joints)

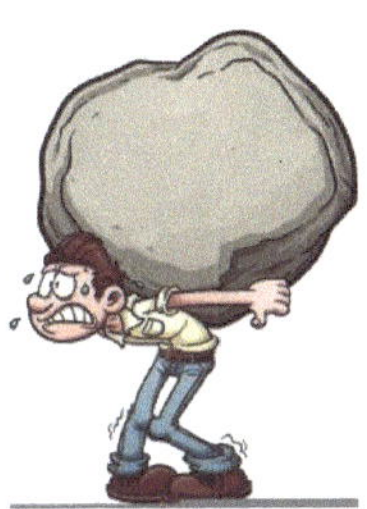

WEIGHT LOSS
First rule of thumb: You MUST burn more calories than you consume.
Second rule: Do not eat simple carbohydrates that turn instantly into fat instead of fuel.
Third rule: If you are toxic, your body will find a way to place fat on your body.
This is where the body stuffs excess toxins. If you are toxic, you will never lose the weight you desire. Ever see these little skinny "Twiggy-type" anorexic-looking girls (I use girls only because I know no guys named Twiggy), and as skinny as they may be, they still have a layer of fat around their middle? This is because they are toxic.

Simple carbohydrates such as bread, pasta, ice-cream, sodas, fried foods, etc. will pack on weight faster than any other foods. Stop them! Freeze a smoothie. Eat vegetable pasta. Drink alkaline water. Bake or grill your foods. And EAT LESS FOOD!

Eating healthy fats, will actually make you lose weight rather than gain. Here's how it works: If you want to burn your own body fat for energy (which is essential if you want to lose weight), you must have low insulin levels. Insulin, tells fat cells to pull fatty acids out of the blood and to keep fat in the fat cells. Whenever you eat carbohydrates, your body floods your bloodstream with insulin. So eating more carbohydrates means less time in fat burning mode, which means more fat accumulation in the fat cells. Which means hunger and weight gain. Eating more fat and fewer carbohydrates means easier fat burning, less hunger, and a better shot at losing weight.

Note: for each ten pounds of fat, your body must make 3,000 to 5,000 miles of capillaries to supply blood to that fat or it would otherwise become gangrenous. When you lose the weight, the body simply reabsorbs the vessels. But, think of how much stress and strain is put on your battery trying to push this much extra fluid through your body.

Potholes

AVOID THE POTHOLES

These can knock your frame out of alignment and put you back up on the rack faster than green grass through a goose.

Plaque deposits- are made up of **cholesterol**, fatty substances, cellular waste products, calcium and fibrin protein that collect in artery pot-holes created from NOT high cholesterol, but poor dietary choices such as "trans fats" like canola oils, corn oils and pretty much any oil overheated to a frying temperature.

Note: Consuming "omega 3" fats instead of trans fats improves the cell's ability to hold a charge.

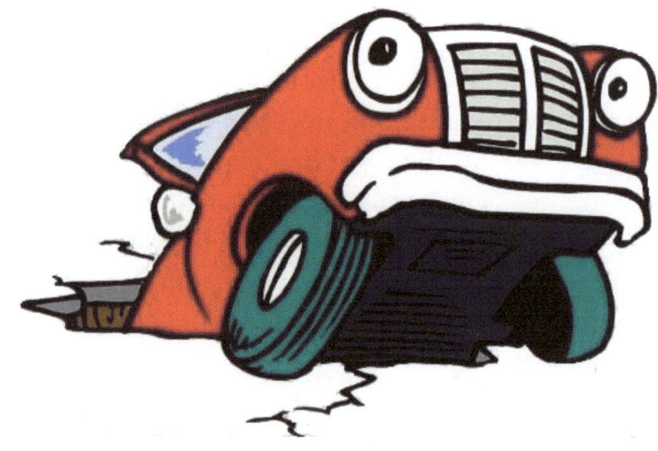

CHAPTR 12   TUNEUP and MAINTENANCE   (Cleanses)

Contents

Oli Filter/Oil Pan Flush

LIVER/GALLBLADDER FLUSH

Removes accumulative toxins from the liver and expels gallstones. Will restore our liver back to nearly as clean as when you were born. Great for removing stored residuals from alcohol consumption, drugs, pharmaceuticals and most ingested toxins.

Fuel System Flush

INTESTINAL FLUSH

Designed to remove 10 and 20-year-old impacted fecal matter from your intestines. Food is not always able to pass through the 30 feet of twists and turns found in the intestines. Your blood visits every portion of your body every three hours, including your intestines. As it passes through, it picks up residue found in the intestines and redistributes it throughout the body. So, your sewer system just grew outside of its designated boundaries and in a short time, your whole body becomes polluted with putrefactive waste and toxins.   **(Better known as "spreadin' the manure.")**

Radiator Flush

MASTER CLEANSE

This is the "waxer-polisher." This cleans your kidneys, tissues, joints, brain eyes, skin and is one of the most wonderful cleanses you can do. However, it does not clean the liver or the intestines. So, if you do this cleanse without the first two, you will simply re-pollute your vehicle once the blood circulates through the intestines.

Again, this is one of the finest cleanses around.

Here's the formula:

1-gallon distilled water

1 cup fresh squeezed lemon juice

¼ to 1 whole cup "Pure" maple syrup. Aunt Jemima won't do!

Mix and drink 8 oz every hour on the hour for 8 hours.

How long do I do this? As long as you like or feel necessary. Raw or pure maple syrup has all the nutrients your body needs in the right proportions. We suggest from 3 to 10 days, depending on the condition and desired results. I have had patients continue for 30 and 40 days. P.S. You eat "no" food during this cleanse. However, we suggest, if you feel light headed, chew up 5 black grapes and spit them out. This will most of the time stop the weird feelings.

With this procedure under our belt, first of all, we can snug our belts up a few notches and secondly, its time to introduce the Formula 6-2-1-1 into our machinery.

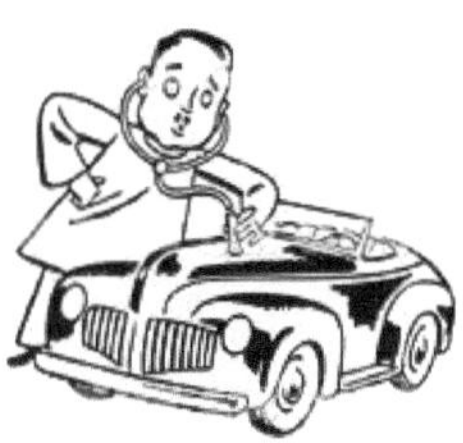

The Paint   (skin)

Your skin is the paint that covers your human vehicle .But it's not just the sack holding all the potatoes in. The skin is also your largest organ, that also serves as part of the body's ventilation and cooling system. But given its many different roles and due to its uniqueness, it has been given its own chapter.

Your paint job is also part of the "Exhaust System" or 5 organs of elimination which consist of the Liver, Kidneys, Intestines, Lungs and Skin. The skin being the largest of the five. Your skin is also part of your dashboard warning lights. If pain is near, if hot or cold is an issue, your paint job warms you of such circumstances. It's a living, breathing paint job. It serves as waterproofing, an insulator shield, a vapor barrier, a protector from damaging sunlight and harmful chemicals and keeps the main-frame computer (the brain) connected to the outside world.

It weighs around 8 pounds and covers approximately 22 square feet. That's eleven feet by eleven feet. (Size may very with each makes and model.)

Now there are a few things we can due to take care of our paint job and keep it remaining lustrous and functioning at peak performance.

Maintenance Program

1 Dry skin brushing- One of the most important steps in protecting and maintaining your paint. Take a dry, natural bristle and scrub you entire body before taking your morning shower. This will eliminate dry skin and surface toxins as well as opening the pores of your paint, assisting in the removal of toxic waste. In addition, the friction produced by the scrubbing will stimulate oxygenation and blood circulation, enhancing overall appearance and skin health.

2 Wax that baby- For an overall shine, an "all-natural" moisturizer will help keep the paint looking new and supple. Almond oil, grape seed oil, Jojoba Oil, Coconut Oil and many other skin oils may be found. Keep bad chemicals off the paint job.

3 Sea salt scrubs are another method of exfoliating dead skin and debris from your paint job. This too increases oxygenation and circulation.

4 Hydration- Water is the number one crucial ingredient for a healthy paint job,

Supplementation:

Collagen	Evening Primrose Oil
Vitamin C. (Antioxidant)	Tulsi (Holy Basil)
B Vitamins. ...	Turmeric
Fatty Acids. ...	

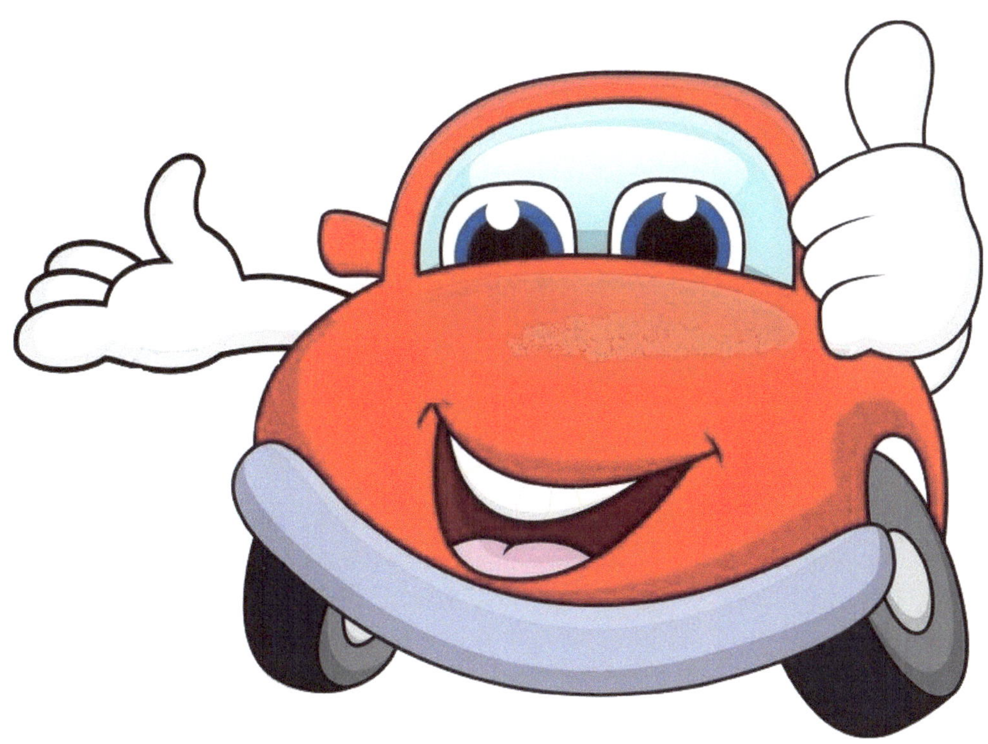

CHAPTER 13 Cooling System (circulatory, water)

Contents

Dehydration

WATER IS ABSOLUTELY CRUCIAL for our health and machinery operations.

Our machine demands at least ½ gallon of water daily. The body weight divided by 2 is the number of ounces of water you need daily.

Dry mouth is one of the last signs the body is dehydrated.

Our blood is 94% of the total body's water supply. If that supply is low, our 94% is also low. This means our vessels shrink to take up the extra left-over room, leading to a major cause of high blood pressure. NOT a deficiency in blood pressure meds.

Not just any fluid will due. Sodas, teas, coffee and other flavored drinks are actually dehydrating, causing you to actually expel more fluid than you take in. Water must be ingested as "water."

Morning sickness is the first sign both the mother and unborn child are dehydrated.

Drink water 30 minutes before each meal. Without water, the hydrolysis (breakdown) of the food particles cannot take place. After the meal, wait 2 ½ hours and drink more water.

When deprived of water, the body will begin to accept there is no water available and will lose the thirst trigger mechanism. This in turn causes the cells in the area of the body most dehydrated, to shrivel up like a prune. This is the sure beginning of chronic disease.

We must have water for cellular function. Water is a hydroelectric generator. It creates voltage. It also transfers nutrients in and toxins out of our cells.

Frequent headaches or leg cramps can be the first signs of dehydration.

Asthma, Heartburn, dyspepsia, Rheumatoid joint pains, migraine headaches and Bulimia are just a few more illnesses triggered by dehydration.

When beginning to increase your water intake, you must also increase your salt intake. Take a pinch of Himalayan or pure sea salt several times a day and allowing it to dissolve on your tongue before drinking. A person has to have enough salt in the body to properly hydrate.

Won't taking salt raise my blood pressure? Here's the answer to that misleading myth. Sodium is not raising your blood pressure, the lack of Calcium, Magnesium and Potassium is. It has been shown that persons on a low-salt diet are more prone to strokes and heart attacks than those on a higher salt diet. When replacing iodized table salt with actual "healthy" salt, you will need to supplement your iodine intake to assure adequate supply for the thyroid gland and production of the hormone thyroxin.

Extra salt in asthma sufferers assists mucus expulsion.

Substitute your coffee and tea drinks with water. You may find your asthma, allergies and high blood pressure disappear.

Persons with heart and kidney disease should up their water intake gradually, insuring their urine output increases with the higher water intake. Within 2 days, if the urine production has not increased, a physician should be consulted.

Constipation screams of DEHYDRATION! Water is the best natural laxative in existence.

So, flush out the radiator of the flavored drinks and replenish the system with good, clean water, preferably Reverse Osmosis and Alkaline. Definitely, not TAP WATER. Any filtering is better than none! Once this is done, a cup of coffee every now and then, will not kill you... or will it?

Cheap formula for alkaline water: If your water tests out at 6.8 pH

1 tsp Baking Soda should bring it up to about 7.4 pH

Add more for more alkalinity and voltage. Don't go over 8.0 pH

for more than a few weeks unless you are ill or extremely acidic>

Check pH's often. 7.4 pH is your goal.

Test with litmus paper.

CHAPTR 14 DRIVING TIPS

Contents

THE DRIVER

Here is the most important part (piece) of the whole machine. This is the one that programs the 70 trillion cells. This is the one that intends the events that manifest into reality. This is the part that must make sure these maintenance procedures are followed. This is YOU! You are owner, driver and boss!

KEEPING THE NEW CAR SMELL (Spirit)

So, let's talk about the essence of your vehicle. This is what keeps it going. This is the newness, the pride and love you have for your vehicle that makes you want to take all these precautions to keep it running smoothly. This is the unseen electricity that courses through the circuitry, that pulsates in the pumps and that propels us through the streets of the cities and flyin' down secluded backwoods dirt roads or just sitting still where we can find quietness and a peacefulness.

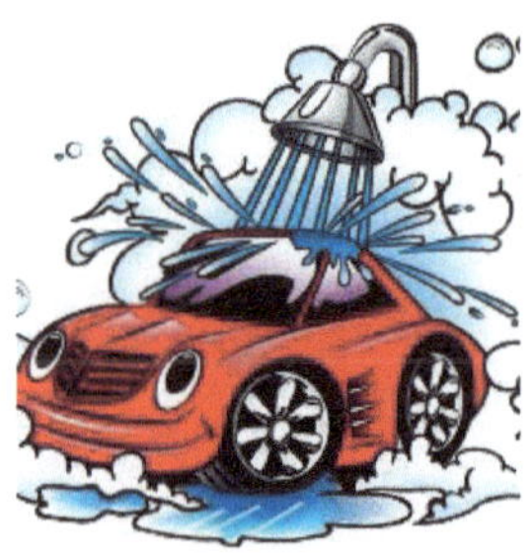

DRIVING SENSIBLY AND SAFELY

You, being the sole operator of your vehicle, want to assure you pay attention and stay aware of what goes into your engine. Read labels. Buy the finest, cleanest foods you can acquire. Avoid alcohol, tobacco, preservatives, food coloring, processed sugar, artificial sweeteners and above all GMO foods. Look for labels stating ORGANIC, NON-GMO, BAKED, etc. Eat everything in moderation. If you do want to occasionally splurge or celebrate, ENJOY IT! Then get back on the wagon, get back in the groove. No harm done. If you fell too far outta the car, do a Master Cleanse for a day.

READ THE ROAD SIGNS

If you feel yourself becoming sluggish, notice what you've been eating. If the condition persists, stop eating and do a gallon of the Master Cleanse formula. If that doesn't fix the problem, you may need an overhaul. In that case a Full Body Detox is in order.

Make sure your iodine level is up to the full line. Your thyroid gland may need a little TLC. There are mineral testing kits available on Amazon.com for checking iodine and 8 more important minerals.

If you feel feverish or feel a cold coming on, add ½ tsp Baking Soda to 4-6 oz of fruit juice. Do this 3 x's a day. This will alkalize your system, killing or detouring the critters. This will also add voltage to your electrical system. This is the "shade tree mechanic's" water alkalizing machine.

Buy some pH strips (litmus paper) and test your pH's regularly. (both urine and saliva) To average the two numbers <u>you must follow this formula</u>: **urine pH + saliva pH + saliva pH divided by 3**, as the saliva number has twice the value of urine. This will tell you the average of your pH. For your overall average, one number is no good without the other. It is best to take the reading at 2:00 pm and 30 minutes to an hour before or after eating food. If this is not possible, rinse your mouth before taking saliva test**.   Be sure to use two different strips for testing the two pH's. It could be most devastional!** If your pH average says you are too acidic (below 7.4 pH) you need more alkaline minerals: potassium, magnesium and calcium. Make sure to use <u>calcium citrate</u> (alkaline) and **not** <u>calcium lactate</u> (acidic).

Note: Never check your pH's first thing in the morning, as they will ALWAYS read acidic. This is when all the junk during the night has been, accumulated, processed and waiting ejection.
(Or, swept up, ground up and waiting for the vacuum to suck 'em up from the shop floor.)

A cheap and quick way to alkalize your body is taking ¼ - ½ tsp Baking Soda in 4 oz. fruit juice or water. If you would like to alkalize your drinking water without spending $300.00 for a machine, you can alkalize your daily water supply in a few short minutes.

Here's the formula:

In 1 gallon of water by adding 1 tsp Baking Soda (B.S.)

Before B.S.	After B.S.
Water pH	New pH
6.0 pH	6.8 pH
7.0 pH	7.8 pH

Use litmus paper or buy an inexpensive pH meter and test your water each time for correct pH. Aim for somewhere between 7.4 pH and 8.0 pH.

Remember: You CAN become TOO alkaline. So, check your pH's every couple of days and try to stay in the total pH average of 7.4 pH. You do this, keep up the iodine level and germs will run from you!

Too acidic means "breeding ground for germs, viruses and bacteria, cold, nervous and workaholic.
Too alkaline means, upper respiratory infections, sinus problems, kidney stones, hot and slow to the point of laziness if not careful.

Interesting tidbit: Your liver produces and uses one drop of natural alcohol per every 60 pounds of body weight, per hour using the sugar in the body. If you know a person that is just so happy-go-lucky, not a care in the world and just nothing matters, it is very possible this person has way too much excess sugar in their body and is literally "drunk" on their own liver-manufactured alcohol. True!

Life is already too short to go and shorten it even more. Enjoy it and by all means DO NOT make eating so stressful you would rather die than eat healthy. Eating should and can be both fun and healthy. Tailor your fuel mixture to your preferences, incorporating as many rules as you are able. Take your time to make the more radical lifestyle changes but make an honest effort in doing so. You'll be doing yourself nothing but a wonderful favor. You can transform your vehicle into anything you desire. Its your choice whether you want to drive an ol' junky jalopy, a luxury vehicle or a high-performance sports car..

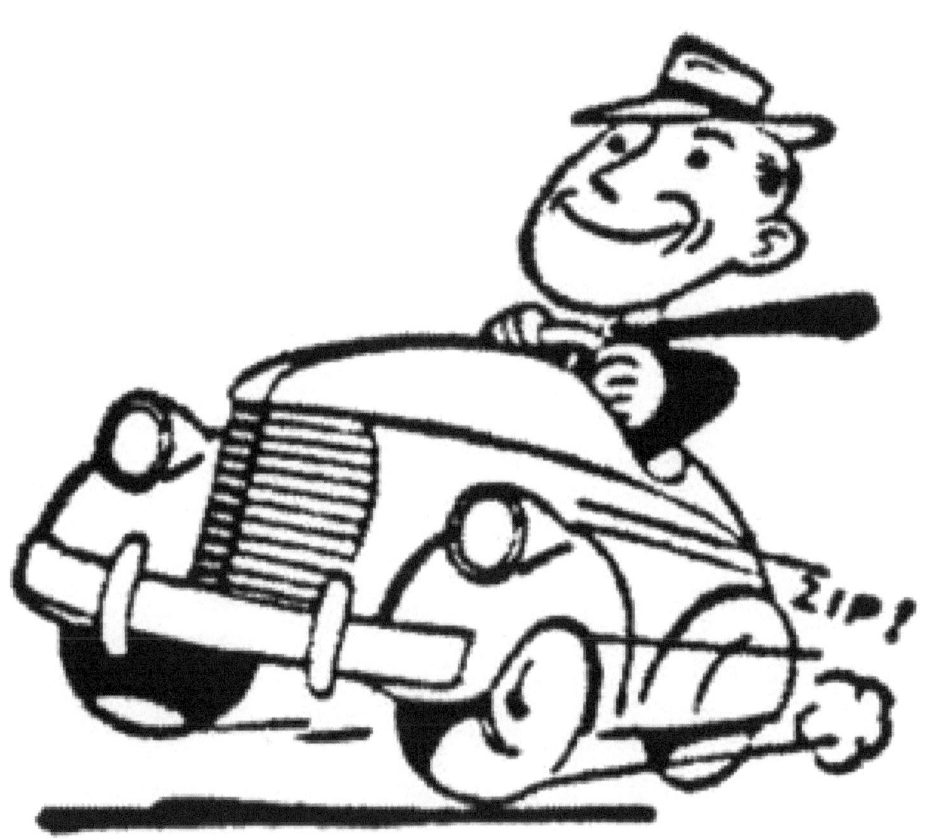

Troubleshooting and Diagnostics

SYMPTOM   **POSSIBILE DIAGNOSIS**

LEG CRAMPS

1. Dehydration
2. Potassium and/or
3. Calcium deficiency

HEARTBURN

1. pH out of range
2. weak enzymes
3. low Hydrochloric Acid

CONSTIPATION

1. Dehydration
2. weak peristalsis
3. excess dairy consumption
4. Too alkaline pH's

DIARRHEA

1. Virus
2. Lactose intolerance
3. Food allergy
4. Fried, greasy food
5. Celiac disease
6. Toxic overload

HEADACHE

1. Dehydration,
2. tight neck
3. trap muscle tightness
4. sinuses blockage or infection
5. tooth infection

ALLERGIES

1. Overactive or "hyper" immune system
2. Poor food choices
3. Immune system over worked and faulty
4. Too much dairy and/or wheat (gluten)

STOMACH ACHE

1. Low gut flora (bacteria)
2. weak digestive enzymes
3. poor food choice
4. grease
5. influenza
6. bacterial infection
7. virus

LOSS OF APPETEITE

1. Virus
2. Stress
3. Psychological
4. Hypothyroidism
5. Anorexia
6. Manganese deficiency

LOWER BACK PAIN

1. Tight muscle
2. spine out of alignment
3. kidney problem
4. dehydration
5. disc injury
6. storing emotions
7. Overweight
8. Manganese deficiency
9. Too much sitting
10. Lack of exercise

ACNE

1. Internal toxins (being pushed out)
2. Chemical reaction
3. Menstrual cycle
4. Stress

HAIR LOSS (non-hereditary)

1. Vitamin D deficiency on of the primary causes
2. Other deficiencies include: A, B's, C, E, iron, selenium zinc
3. Alopecia

BRITTLE OR CRACKING FINGER NAILS

1. Deficiencies: B Vitamins, Folic Acid, Omega 3, Vit. C, calcium
2. Thyroid disorder
3. Frequent manicures
4. Too much nail polish
5. Too much nail polish remover
6. Fungal infection
7. If ridges, Biotin deficiency.

CHAPPED SKIN ON HANDS   (CRACKS IN THE PAINT JOB)

1. Lack of silica
2. Lack of correct fats in skin
3. Cold weather

ITCHING PALMS AND SOLES OF FEET

1. Deficiencies in potassium, Sulphur and chlorine

ALWAYS COLD

1. body pH's too acid (not enough friction)
2. thyroid underactive (hypothyroid)
3. low iodine levels
4. Low iron levels

ALWAYS HOT

1. dehydrated
2. pH's too alkaline (too much friction)
3. hyperthyroid
4. menopause
5. caffeine
6. diabetes
7. blood vessels not dilating,
8. overweight

JOINT PAIN

1. Dehydration
2. crystalized acid deposits
3. overweight
4. join injury
5. gout

6. body pH's too acidic
7. bursitis
8. arthritis,
9. inflammation
10. Organic sodium deficiency (not iodized table salt)

TIRED

1. Toxic
2. Low thyroid
3. sleep deprivation
4. adrenal failure
5. anemia
6. B-12 deficiency
7. low blood pressure
8. too much blood pressure medicine
9. chronic fatigue,
10. urinary tract infection
11. Herpes
12. Poor food choices
13. Vitamin/mineral deficiencies and out of balance

THINKING FOGGY

1. Dehydration
2. low electrolyte levels
3. toxic
4. dementia
5. poor nutrition
6. low blood sugar
7. poor blood circulation to brain
8. sleep deprivation
9. endocrine imbalances
10. medication side effects
11. Radiation exposure from cell phone. Too close to head during use. (keep 6-12" from head. Use speaker.)

MEMORY LOSS

1. B-12 deficiency
2. hypothyroidism
3. low electrolytes
4. dementia
5. trauma
6. Alzheimer's

   7. alcoholism

   8. medication (especially Statin drugs)

   9. emotional disorders

  10. Brain tumor (the most extreme)

  11. Low iron causes low oxygen

PAIN IN CHEST

1. Angina (stress)
2. C7 cervical vertebrae out
3. intercostal muscle strain
4. heart attack
5. peptic ulcer
6. GERD
7. injured ribs
8. inflammation of rib tendons
9. dehydration
10. Gas

BURNING PAIN IN NAVEL

1. appendicitis
2. peptic ulcer
3. digestive problem
4. cramp- like may be diarrhea or constipation
5. pinched nerve

PAIN IN LEFT SIDE

1. diverticulitis
2. gas
3. indigestion
4. kidney stones
5. hernia,
6. shingles (if burning)

Women only-

1. menstrual cramps
2. endometriosis
3. ovarian-cyst
4. ectopic pregnancy (fertilized egg implanted before
5. reaching the uterus.)

Men only-

1. inguinal hernia
2. rotated testicle

NAUSEA AFTER EATING

1. Food poisoning
2. gastritis
3. ulcer
4. gallbladder issue
5. bulimia
6. weak digestive enzymes
7. food allergies

NAUSEA CONSTANT

1. Toxic
2. dehydration
3. poor or slow digestion
4. weak digestive or lack of digestive enzymes
5. ulcer
6. stomach cancer
7. Spleen complications
8. If, when excited, potassium deficiency is suggested

SEIZURES

1. dehydration
2. food or chemical allergy
3. Aspartame sensitivity
4. RF (radio frequency) sensitivity
5. abnormality in brain or brain chemistry
6. head trauma
7. cell phone too close to head
8. If epileptic, deficiency in manganese

SLEEPLESSNESS

1. Adrenal failure
2. high cortisol level
3. drug and/or alcohol abuse
4. caffeine
5. Too much Red-Bull stimulants
6. sleep aide addiction
7. stress
8. chromic pain
9. hyperthyroidism
10. asthma
11. sleep apnea

12. excessive RF signals in bedroom
13. More restless sitting or lying, than standing, potassium deficiency is probable.

WEIGHT GAIN

1. Toxic
2. Consuming more calories than burning
3. poor dietary habits
4. hypothyroidism
5. too many simple carbs (bread, pasta, etc.)
6. dehydration
7. stress
8. anxiety
9. depression (these previous three all
10. lead to eating poorly and too much)
11. menopause or pre-menopausal
12. lack of exercise

WEIGHT LOSS

1. over active thyroid
2. inflammatory bowel disease
3. anxiety
4. burning more calories than consuming
5. diabetes
6. endocarditis (infection of the inner lining of heart)
7. drug abuse

ULCER

1. Stress
2. poor dietary habits
3. too much grease
4. too acidic
5. too many acidic drinks; coffee, tea, sodas
6. medication (especially NSAID's like Advil and Aleve) and other non-steroidal anti-inflammatory drugs
7. too much aspirin
8. too many spicy foods.

RESTLESS LEGS

1. Toxic
2. Too acidic (Acid energy travels downward)

3. Too much caffeine

4. Drug abuse

5. Nicotine excess

6. If hot feet, too much energy arrive at intersection
   all at the same time.

COMPACT CARS Children and smaller models

BABY CRYING EXCESSIVELY

1. Colicky
2. Too much cow's milk
3. Hungry
4. Teething
5. Wants attention (needs held)
6. Needs changing
8. Too hot or cold
9. Doesn't feel well (check engine temp.)
10. Magnesium deficiency. Crying uses magnesium up.
    (Also uses it up in the parents who can't get enough
    sleep. Supplement them as well)

ATTENTION DEFICIT

1. Too much sugar
2. Mind not being stimulated adequately
3. Manganese deficiency
4. Insufficient nutrition

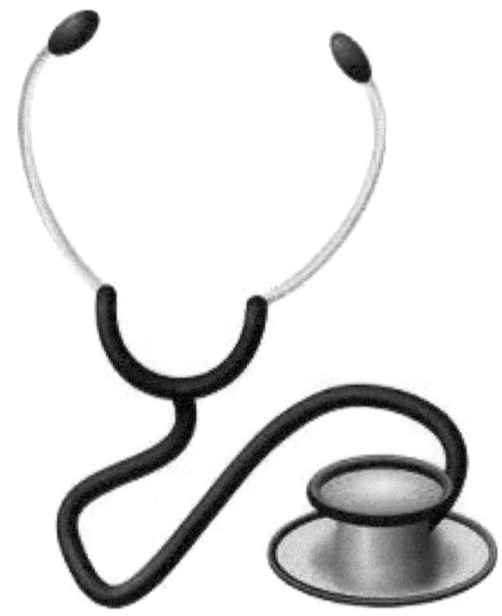

HIGH PERFORMANCE SHOP

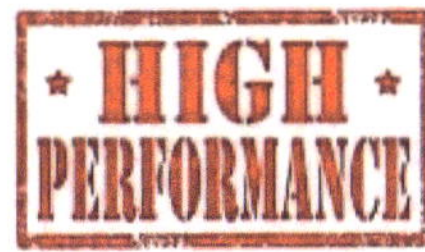

Products and where to purchase:

FULL BODY CLEANSE KIT-Castle in the Clouds L.L.C.   (There is no finer or more thorough.)
OMNI-IMMMUNE- Castle in the Clouds L.L.C. (Kills all mold, yeast, fungi, viruses and bacteria.)
INTRA-MAX- Castle in the Clouds L.L.C.   (415 nutrients, 100% absorption.)
LIPO-SOMAL GLUTATHIONE- www.Redi-sorb.com or www. Amazon.com
LIPO-SOMAL VITAMIN C- www.LivonLabs.com or www.Amazon .com
D-OXYGENATOR- Castle in the Clouds Health Center L.L.C.

   In home portable oxygen delivery system. Relax in your bathtub or hot tub with your own personal oxygen machine. Delivers concentrated atomic oxygen, saturating every cell and interstitial space in your body with powerful, healing oxygen. No other modality can provide as much oxygen to your body as the D-Oxygenator. More info available upon request. Special Reader's Price

SUPERCHARGERS   (Brain boosters)

   Phosphatidylserine- It supports human cognitive functions, including the formation of short-term memory, the consolidation of long-term memory, the ability to create new memories, the ability to retrieve memories, the ability to learn and recall information, the ability to focus attention and concentrate, the ability to reason and solve problems, language skills, and the ability to communicate. It also supports locomotor functions, especially rapid reactions and reflexes.

   NADH- Nicotinamide adenine dinucleotide, is the active form of vitamin B-3. It is normally produced in your body. Improves nerve signaling in the brain, which may diminish symptoms associated with Parkinson's or Alzheimer's disease' I have seen it work wonders for firing up the brain. It must be used in conjunction with the following. (ATP)

   ATP- Adenosine triphosphate is a cell food, able to boost blood flow along with increasing stamina while exercising. The reason it is listed here is because it must be used in conjunction with NADH for the full effectiveness of the NADH to be achieved.

   5 HTP- mood elevator increases serotonin levels in your body, which may improve symptoms of depression, especially when used in conjunction with the amino acid L-Theanine.

   DOPA- improve mental performance, including focus, attention, creativity, and learning. See a reduction in brain fog and an increase in clear thinking and cognitive function - Increase in physical and athletic balance, as well as motor function

   EFA's- Essential fatty acids appear here again because they are extremely important in brain functions such a neurotransmissions, memory functions and increased brain activity. It may take 2 to 3 months to build up to a noticeable effect, but when they do, look out! **Dosage:** 1200 I.U.- 2 or 3 x's a day.

   L-Tryptophan- amino acid for depression.

   L-Theanine- amino acid for anxiety. This is also the fastest way to lower cortisol levels from over stimulated or adrenal failure. Adrenal failure leads to extremely levels of cortisol. If you have sleep deprivation due to adrenal overload, you probably have 85% more cortisol in your bloodstream than you should have. Until this is lowered, you will never achieve a good night's sleep.

For information ,pricing and/or purchasing products, or
to schedule a personal consultation with Dr. Mark, contact:
Castle in the Clouds Health Center
castlesexton@hotmail.com
or call
573-317-1912

Castle in the Clouds L.L.C. provides a wide-range of very successful alternative treatment therapies including in-house and outpatient services.

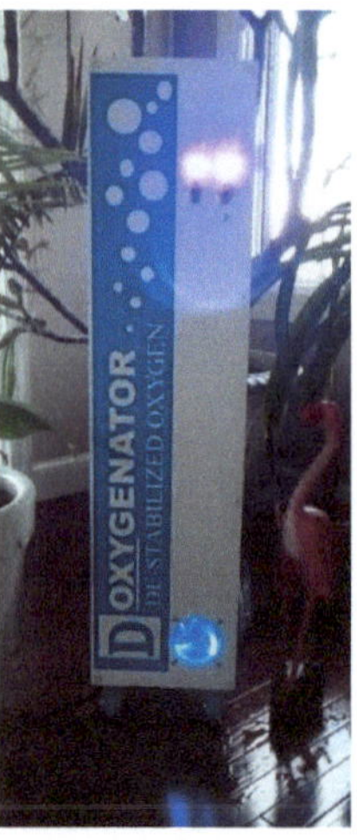

The D-Oxygenator

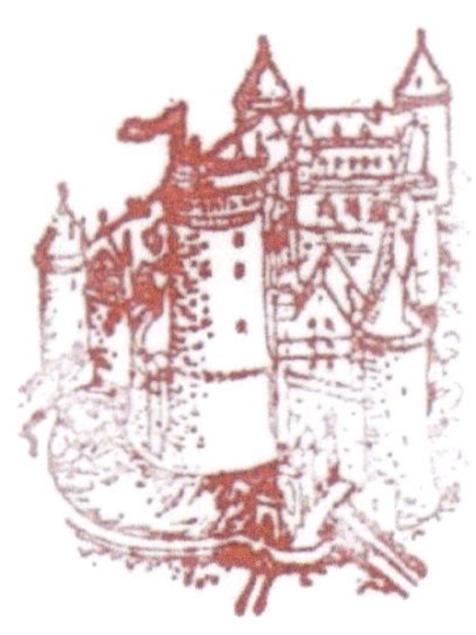

ENGINE SPECS AND FLUID LEVELS

ENGINE SPECIFICATIONS

Tire pressure (Blood pressure)	systolic 60-90 diastolic 90-130
RPM (Pulse rate)	60-100 BPM (beats per minute)
Temperature	97.8-99.1
Exhaust (Breathing rate)	12-18 BPM (breaths per minute)

FLUIDS AND ADDITIVES

Water	½ gallon daily (minimum)
Calcium	1 gram (1000 mg) a day
Magnesium	400-800 mg a day (also a great sleep aid if taken before bed)
Potassium	2000-4000 mg a day (with adequate water, stops leg cramps)
Salt	2-3 grams a day (+ cal., mag, pot. and water)
Liquid Multi Vit/Min supp.	Intra-Max is my suggestion (415 nutrients) plus the above

LUBRICATION POINTS

(Use a good grade EFA oil. Cold Pressed)
ALL JOINTS
BRAIN
NERVOUS SYSTEM

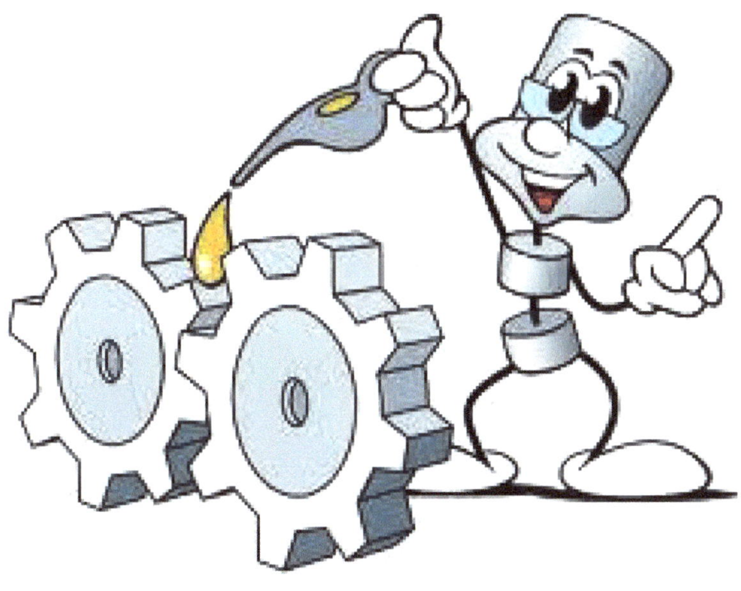

pH and VOLTAGE CHART

CELL VOLTAGE	CELL pH's	
-50	7.88	MAKES NEW CELLS
-45	7.79	
-40	7.70	
-35	7.61	NORMAL FOR KIDS
-30	7.53	
-25	7.44	NORMAL FOR ADULTS
-20	7.35	
-15	7.26	TIRED
-10	7.18	SICK
-5	7.09	
0 neutral pH	7.00	POLARITY BEGINS CHANGING (most drinking water)
+5	6.91	
+10	6.83	
+20	6.85	BREEDING GROUND FOR GERMS
+30	6.48	CANCER OCCURS
+57.14	6.0	ADVANCED CANCER
+68.57	5.8	STAGE 4 CANCER
+142.86	4.5	DEAD CELL
+228.57	3.0	WINE
+257.14	2.5	SODA/COFFEE

Note: Remember most drinking water is kept at 7.0 pH. Drinking an 8oz soda, you need to drink 32- 8oz glasses of 10 pH water to neutralize the cola back to 7.0 pH. Soda and coffee are twice as acidic as a dead cell.

Personal note to the Readers:

" I hope you found my Human Repair Manual to be fun as well as informative, helpful and easy to understand. On a final note: If you don't practice it yet, meditation is one of the finest practices to balance your engine and enhance its overall performance. It will reduce stress and is one of the best anti-aging techniques in existence. Look for my up-coming books and CD's on this subject. Thanks for reading and please, suggest this to your friends."

Dr. Mark